The Mediterranean Diet for Beginners

The Complete Guide with More than 100 Delicious Recipes, and Tips for Success!

By

Alexander Sandler

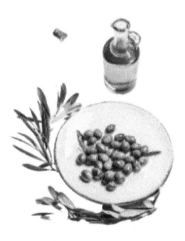

TABLE OF CONTENT

INTRODUCTION

The Mediterranean diet does not explicitly exclude any food group; it simply promotes better food choices such as replacing bad fats with good fats, red meat with seafood, etc. It encourages foods that are as close to their natural state as possible. The Mediterranean diet is one the easiest diets to follow and one of the best diets for a wide range of chronic diseases. Mediterranean diet has been shown to lower the risk of diabetes, cardiovascular disease, and cancer. The Mediterranean diet can help you shed unwanted pounds and slow the aging process by five to ten years. And you know, what makes the eating habits of the Italians and Greeks such a brilliant diet plan is that it's not just about the food, but an entire lifestyle! Over the decades, the Mediterranean diet has seen a slow rise in the Western world. Many Western countries were slow to pick it up, but they realized they had discovered the key to the Elixir of Life once they did. Not only has the Mediterranean diet helped people rely on a healthy, wholesome diet, but it has helped them lose weight, boost their immune systems, improve their vitality, and even contribute to healthy skin. In other words, the Mediterranean diet helped people feel good and look good. The combination of benefits changed people's perceptions of what they should eat and challenged their eating habits.

For example, many people often skip breakfast because they think having a meal in the morning adds more weight to their bodies. However, the Mediterranean diet does not skip breakfast. On the contrary, it considers breakfasting the most important meal of the day. Countries that have relied on the Mediterranean diet had seen its benefits long before scientific research was conducted. They did not have any study conducted to guide them to a particular dietary pattern or food content. Essentially, the diet has been refined over the millennia as new cooking methods were introduced. But adherence to a healthy form of the diet has remained, regardless of the diet's age.

This diet is the typical diet of the people of the Mediterranean area. It has been proven to be healthier than typical American and British diets. This diet contains lots of fresh fruits, vegetables, and fish. It also allows you to consume whole grains instead of refined white rice like other diets. The Mediterranean diet is considered a low-glycemic eating pattern, which means it does not raise blood sugar levels. It has many vitamins and minerals that help support a healthy heart and robust immune system.

This book was written specifically for people who want to get into this healthy way of eating. It will teach you how the Mediterranean diet can change your life forever!

For centuries, people have been cutting back on unhealthy foods and adding more healthy foods to their diets. Yet, for some reason, this good habit seems to have stopped before it even began. Not anymore. In "Mediterranean Diet Meal Preparation," you'll learn the secrets to losing belly fat: and getting your body in better shape.

This book will help you on how you can:

Get healthy with new food choices. Get more energy.

Lose belly fat: without diets; by taking advantage of homemade meal preparation methods. Find healthy alternatives for traditional desserts. We are getting the proper nutrients.

The Mediterranean could be considered a decorative and beautiful plant. In the Mediterranean region, there are so many palm trees that give the area a resort-like atmosphere. However, the plant has gained popularity in recent years because it has several health benefits. This diet emphasizes foods that are fresh, whole, unprocessed, and minimally altered. Benefits of eating the Mediterranean way include a lower risk of heart disease, cancer, stroke, depression, obesity, and diabetes.

MEDITERRANEAN DIET AND IT'S THE BENEFITS

In this nutrition and health-conscious world, medical scientists, nutritionists, and health scientists continue to search for healthy options and lifestyle changes that can ensure health and longevity along with agility. There is an emerging consensus among health experts that a diet with fiber and a balanced amount of protein, healthy fats, and minerals can lead to optimal health and healthy living. It can control cardiovascular disease, diabetes, cancer, and stroke and help maintain a healthy weight. The Mediterranean diet has all of these attributes. Its ingredients are rich in plants, healthy fats, fruits, whole grains, healthy meats, and more. It has all the elements that are essential for a healthy diet. There have been claims about its positive effect on health and physical well-being.

A study conducted on 25,000 women over 12 years determined that those who consume the Mediterranean diet have a 25% lower chance of having cardiovascular disease. This positive change is decreased inflammation and blood glucose levels and a better body mass index.

There is little saturated fat with a high amount of monounsaturated fat, protein, and dietary fiber. Olive oil has an important health element which is oleic acid. It is highly beneficial for human heart health. It has the European Food Safety Authority Panel's approval on Dietetic Products, Nutrition, and Allergies. It has been said that its polyphenols protect against the oxidation of blood lipids. This happens because of the priority given to olive oil, which has oleic acid that helps maintain normal LDL in the blood and control cardiovascular disease. The American Heart Association has also stated that consuming olive oil can help maintain cardiovascular health. If you follow this diet, your refined bread, processed foods, and unhealthy meats will be reduced. The diet also recommends replacing hard liquor with red wine. It is scientifically already proven that the Mediterranean diet can reduce the risk of cardiovascular disease.

This diet has a high fiber content. This reduces the blood glucose level and controls the causes that develop type 2 diabetes. This fiber makes you feel full and keeps cravings under control. This also helps in keeping weight under control and reduces constipation and helps in regulating bowel movement.

Maintaining a healthy weight is the main point in good health. It becomes easy to maintain an ideal weight when you follow a diet rich in fruits and vegetables. When combined with a physical routine, it becomes easy to maintain a healthy weight. This can help reduce obesity as well. Besides, maintaining an ideal weight can give us multiple health benefits.

Through comprehensive research, it has been found that regular, monitored consumption of the Mediterranean diet can minimize the risk of death from cancer by five to six percent. This was confirmed in a study conducted on cancer patients in 2017. It was also found that the Mediterranean diet can decrease the chances of cancer.

Stress is the key factor that negatively affects life today. The Mediterranean diet can be a relaxant in this case. In various studies, a sincere adherence to the Mediterranean diet can control the deterioration of cognitive abilities. It does this by improving good cholesterol, blood sugar levels, and overall blood vessel health. This, as a result, reduces the risk of dementia or Alzheimer's disease.

With whole vegetables, fruits, and nuts, the Mediterranean diet is rich in antioxidants, vitamins, and other nutrients. This protects cells from damage that would otherwise occur from oxidative stress. As a result, it reduces the risk of Parkinson's disease by fifty percent. Adhering to this diet can also lower the causes of depression and give you a healthier state of mind.

A study conducted by food scientists on women who had chances of stroke in the UK noted that when they followed the Mediterranean diet very strictly, it reduced their chances of getting a stroke by twenty percent. By the way, this was not the case in men. Clinical research is underway to observe its effect on the male gender as well.

The National Institute on Aging funded a small study on aging that was published in 2018. The review showed that brain scans of 70 people showed that people who adhered strictly to the Mediterranean diet showed no signs of aging, while those who had a preference for other forms of diet had a pattern of plaques that added to the adverse effect of aging. This shows that the Mediterranean diet adds longevity to human life and gives lasting health. The lungs play an important role in oxygenating our bodies, but their ability to inhale deteriorates as we age. Whole grains, dairy products, and fish can improve the lungs' ability to function better. Besides, those who remain disciplined and consistent in following the Mediterranean diet have a 22-29% lower chance of losing their hearing.

It is an obvious fact that the Mediterranean diet has ample amounts of nutrients. If we consume this diet, it helps prevent muscle damage, increases muscle strength, and improves agility. This improves the efficiency of the brain. This means that this diet's consumers have better thinking and learning abilities, better memory, and concentration.

This diet is very beneficial for kidney patients and those who have had a kidney transplant. In some studies, it has been found that diet can reduce the risk of kidney dysfunction. It can also minimize graft failure by 32 percent and graft loss by 26 percent in kidney transplant patients.

If a person develops inflammatory bowel disease such as hemorrhoids, the Mediterranean diet can cause a cure. After studies and case studies, it has been found that consumers of this diet are 57% less likely to develop Crohn's disease.

The benefits are manifold, and nutritionists are still counting.

HOW TO START

The best way to cause change is to initiate it. But the bigger question is how to get started. The situation is much better if what we need to begin has multiple benefits. The Mediterranean diet falls into this category, where the benefits outweigh the limitations it can impose on our lifestyle.

If you feel that it is challenging to change your diet, you can choose alternatives that work well and switch to a healthier option. Here are some ways that can help you make the switch to the Mediterranean diet.

It's good to start by keeping vegetables and fruits at the top of the priority list and putting sausage and pepperoni on the back burner in your salad dressing. You can start by giving a plate of tomato slices a try. You should give it just a drizzle of olive oil and some crushed feta cheese. Soups, crudité dishes, and salads can be great starters.

Skipping breakfast may seem effective, but it can put an extra load on your system to keep you going. On the other hand, whole grains, fruits, and other fiber-rich foods can be an effective way to start your day. Plus, they'll keep you full and your cravings at bay.

Replace the usual calorie-laden sweets like cakes, ice cream, pastries, etc., with fruits like apples, grapes, fresh figs, or strawberries. This will make you digest better and stay lighter. A refreshing feeling will work as motivation and keep you adhering to this magical diet.

If you pop in for a change, it may never happen. There is a famous saying, "A journey of a thousand miles begins with a single step." This is quite applicable to switching to the Mediterranean diet. You can start with small steps like skipping with olive oil and eating more vegetables and fruits in your salad. Replace your snacks with fruit. Similarly, other heavy dishes can be replaced with vegetables.

Choose skim milk or milk with 2% fat instead of whole milk. This will make you feel lighter and healthier. As a result, it will work as a motivating factor to opt for the Mediterranean diet. The change in energy level and diet will work as a trigger and driving force.

It is said that if it is easy, it is doable. The most affordable thing is to use whole grains instead of refined grains. Your choice should be whole-grain bread and not white bread that is made from refined flour. Similarly, brown rice or wild rice should replace white rice. Sometimes it is difficult to choose authentic whole grains. However, it's easy because the Oldways Whole Grain Council has developed a black and gold stamp to select quality over pasta.

Ancient grains or whole grains are an essential part of the Mediterranean diet. There is a huge variety of these grains. These are amaranth, faro, millet, spelled, and the credible Egyptian Kamut; another is teff, which is similar in size to poppy seeds. You can try one seed at a time. Slowly and steadily, you can move on to more options. Each seed has its flavor and texture. The good news is that these whole grains have become quite popular and are pretty standard. In fact, they are now available in mainstream restaurants as well. This means that you can try them and then make them part of your diet.

If you decide to do so, you should have at least six servings a day. Half should be whole grains. It may be worrisome for some because of the carbs, but you can throw your caution to the wind because it will indeed cause long-term benefits. You shouldn't overlook the fact that rapid weight loss may not be healthy. So, whole wheat in the Mediterranean diet is the best option.

You may not be able to change your current diet with the Mediterranean diet at once. So, try a meal of vegetables, whole grains, and beans. Use spices and herbs to add a palatable punch.

If you are protein-conscious and remain preoccupied with your diet, your dependence on meat could end by making room for lentils in your diet. Lentils are high sources of protein and also have a lot of fiber. Beans have an advantage because they have a lot of antioxidants. What motivation!

Fill your pantry with beneficial ingredients. These ingredients should be easy to use. Some of them can be popular protein sources like lentils, chickpeas, and beans. Lentils require only 25 minutes of cooking time, with no overnight soaking required. As for canned chickpeas and beans, just rinse them; then, you can put them in soups, burgers, salads, sandwiches, and more.

Giving up meat altogether can be a challenge, but you can give it a start by taking meat in small proportions. Use cut pieces of chicken or slices of lean meat. You can fry your dish and avoid frying. This will keep it less impregnated with oil and more nutritious. This is good news for fish eaters, as when they are on the Mediterranean diet, they can eat two servings of salmon, sardines, and tuna, which are essential to the Mediterranean diet. There may be a risk of mercury, but in the opinion of American nutritionists, the benefits outweigh the risk. The variety of fish mentioned here has relatively less mercury.

Dairy products can be a great source of protein. A Greek yogurt is a great option, but it should be consumed in moderation.

In short, the Mediterranean diet is a healthy option with a wide range of tasty choices. If you start with a simple approach, taking small steps at a time, making minor changes to your eating plan, you can go a long way.

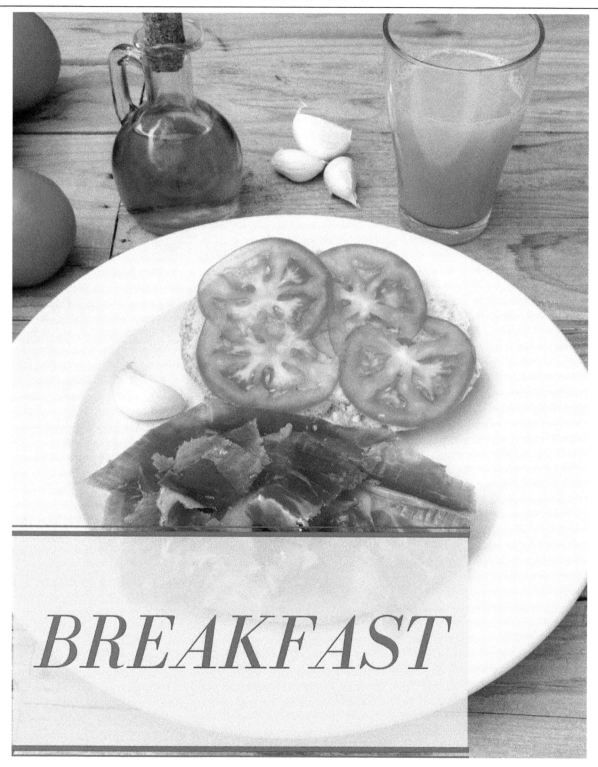

BREAKFAST

1) COUSCOUS PEARL SALAD

Cooking Time: 10 Minutes   **Servings: 6**

Ingredients:

- ✓ lemon juice, 1 large lemon
- ✓ 1/3 cup extra-virgin olive oil
- ✓ 1 tsp dill weed
- ✓ 1 tsp garlic powder
- ✓ salt
- ✓ pepper
- ✓ 2 cups Pearl Couscous
- ✓ 2 tbsp extra virgin olive oil
- ✓ 2 cups grape tomatoes, halved
- ✓ water as needed
- ✓ 1/3 cup red onions, finely chopped
- ✓ ½ English cucumber, finely chopped
- ✓ 1 15-ounce can chickpeas
- ✓ 1 14-ounce can artichoke hearts, roughly chopped
- ✓ ½ cup pitted Kalamata olives
- ✓ 15-20 pieces fresh basil leaves, roughly torn and chopped
- ✓ 3 ounces fresh mozzarella

Directions:

- ❖ Start by preparing the vinaigrette by mixing all Ingredients: in a bowl. Set aside.
- ❖ Heat olive oil in a medium-sized heavy pot over medium heat.
- ❖ Add couscous and cook until golden brown.
- ❖ Add 3 cups of boiling water and cook the couscous according to package instructions.
- ❖ Once done, drain in a colander and put it to the side.
- ❖ In a large mixing bowl, add the rest of the Ingredients: except the cheese and basil.
- ❖ Add the cooked couscous, basil, and mix everything well.
- ❖ Give the vinaigrette a gentle stir and whisk it into the couscous salad. Mix well.
- ❖ Adjust/add seasoning as desired.
- ❖ Add mozzarella cheese.
- ❖ Garnish with some basil.
- ❖ Enjoy!

Nutrition: Calories: 578, Total Fat: 25.3g, Saturated Fat: 4.6, Cholesterol: 8 mg, Sodium: 268 mg, Total Carbohydrate: 70.1g, Dietary Fiber: 17.5 g, Total Sugars: 10.8 g, Protein: 23.4 g, Vitamin D: 0 mcg, Calcium: 150 mg, Iron: 6 mg, Potassium: 1093 mg

2) TOMATO MUSHROOM EGG CUPS

Cooking Time: 5 Minutes   **Servings: 4**

Ingredients:

- ✓ 4 eggs
- ✓ 1/2 cup tomatoes, chopped
- ✓ 1/2 cup mushrooms, chopped
- ✓ 2 tbsp fresh parsley, chopped
- ✓ 1/4 cup half and half
- ✓ 1/2 cup cheddar cheese, shredded
- ✓ Pepper
- ✓ Salt

Directions:

- ❖ In a bowl, whisk the egg with half and half, pepper, and salt.
- ❖ Add tomato, mushrooms, parsley, and cheese and stir well.
- ❖ Pour egg mixture into the four small jars and seal jars with lid.
- ❖ Pour 1 1/2 cups of water into the instant pot then place steamer rack in the pot.
- ❖ Place jars on top of the steamer rack.
- ❖ Seal pot with lid and cook on high for 5 minutes.
- ❖ Once done, release pressure using quick release. Remove lid.
- ❖ Serve and enjoy.

Nutrition: Calories: 146;Fat: 10.g;Carbohydrates: 2.5 g;Sugar: 1.2 g;Protein: 10 g;Cholesterol: 184 mg

3) BREAKFAST MEDITERRANEAN-STYLE SALAD

Cooking Time: 10 Minutes   **Servings: 2**

Ingredients:

- ✓ 4 eggs (optional)
- ✓ 10 cups arugula
- ✓ 1/2 seedless cucumber, chopped
- ✓ 1 cup cooked quinoa, cooled
- ✓ 1 large avocado
- ✓ 1 cup natural almonds, chopped
- ✓ 1/2 cup mixed herbs like mint and dill, chopped
- ✓ 2 cups halved cherry tomatoes and/or heirloom tomatoes cut into wedges
- ✓ Extra virgin olive oil
- ✓ 1 lemon
- ✓ Sea salt, to taste
- ✓ Freshly ground black pepper, to taste

Directions:

- ❖ Cook the eggs by soft-boiling them - Bring a pot of water to a boil, then reduce heat to a simmer. Gently lower all the eggs into water and allow them to simmer for 6 minutes. Remove the eggs from water and run cold water on top to stop the cooking, process set aside and peel when ready to use
- ❖ In a large bowl, combine the arugula, tomatoes, cucumber, and quinoa
- ❖ Divide the salad among 2 containers, store in the fridge for 2 days
- ❖ To Serve: Garnish with the sliced avocado and halved egg, sprinkle herbs and almonds over top. Drizzle with olive oil, season with salt and pepper, toss to combine. Season with more salt and pepper to taste, a squeeze of lemon juice, and a drizzle of olive oil

Nutrition: Calories:2;Carbs: 18g;Total Fat: 16g;Protein: 10g

4) CARROT OATMEAL BREAKFAST

Cooking Time: 10 Minutes   **Servings: 2**

Ingredients:

- ✓ 1 cup steel-cut oats
- ✓ 1/2 cup raisins
- ✓ 1/2 tsp ground nutmeg
- ✓ 1/2 tsp ground cinnamon
- ✓ 2 carrots, grated
- ✓ 2 cups of water
- ✓ 2 cups unsweetened almond milk
- ✓ 1 tbsp honey

Directions:

- ❖ Spray instant pot from inside with cooking spray.
- ❖ Add all ingredients into the instant pot and stir well.
- ❖ Seal pot with lid and cook on high for 10 minutes.
- ❖ Once done, release pressure using quick release. Remove lid.
- ❖ Stir and serve.

Nutrition: Calories: 3;Fat: 6.6 g;Carbohydrates: 73.8 g;Sugar: 33.7 g;Protein: 8.1 g;Cholesterol: 0 mg

5) ARBORIO RICE RUM-RAISIN PUDDING

Cooking Time: 4 Hours   **Servings: 2**

Ingredients:

- ✓ ¾ cup Arborio rice
- ✓ 1 can evaporated milk
- ✓ ½ cup raisins
- ✓ ¼ tsp nutmeg, grated
- ✓ 1½ cups water
- ✓ 1/3 cup sugar
- ✓ ¼ cup dark rum
- ✓ sea salt or plain salt

Directions:

- ❖ Start by mixing rum and raisins in a bowl and set aside.
- ❖ Then, heat the evaporated milk and water in a saucepan and then simmer.
- ❖ Now, add sugar and stir until dissolved.
- ❖ Finally, convert this milk mixture into a slow cooker and stir in rice and salt. Cook on low heat for hours.
- ❖ Now, stir in the raisin mixture and nutmeg and let sit for 10 minutes.
- ❖ Serve warm.

Nutrition: Calories: 3, Total Fat: 10.1g, Saturated Fat: 5.9, Cholesterol: 36 mg, Sodium: 161 mg, Total Carbohydrate: 131.5 g, Dietary Fiber: 3.3 g, Total Sugars: 54.8 g, Protein: 14.4 g, Vitamin D: 0 mcg, Calcium: 372 mg, Iron: 2 mg, Potassium: 712 mg

6) MEDITERRANEAN-STYLE QUINOA WITH FETA EGG MUFFINS

Cooking Time: 30 Minutes   **Servings: 12**

Ingredients:

- ✓ 8 eggs
- ✓ 1 cup cooked quinoa
- ✓ 1 cup crumbled feta cheese
- ✓ 1/4 tsp salt
- ✓ 2 cups baby spinach finely chopped
- ✓ 1/2 cup finely chopped onion
- ✓ 1 cup chopped or sliced tomatoes, cherry or grape tomatoes
- ✓ 1/2 cup chopped and pitted Kalamata olives
- ✓ 1 tbsp chopped fresh oregano
- ✓ 2 tsp high oleic sunflower oil plus optional extra for greasing muffin tins

Directions:

- ❖ Pre-heat oven to 350 degrees F
- ❖ Prepare 1silicone muffin holders on a baking sheet, or grease a 12-cup muffin tin with oil, set aside
- ❖ In a skillet over medium heat, add the vegetable oil and onions, sauté for 2 minutes
- ❖ Add tomatoes, sauté for another minute, then add spinach and sauté until wilted, about 1 minute
- ❖ Remove from heat and stir in olives and oregano, set aside
- ❖ Place the eggs in a blender or mixing bowl and blend or mix until well combined
- ❖ Pour the eggs in to a mixing bowl (if you used a blender) then add quinoa, feta cheese, veggie mixture, and salt, and stir until well combined
- ❖ Pour mixture in to silicone cups or greased muffin tins, dividing equally, and bake for 30 minutes, or until eggs have set and muffins are a light golden brown
- ❖ Allow to cool completely
- ❖ Distribute among the containers, store in fridge for 2-3 days
- ❖ To Serve: Heat in the microwave for 30 seconds or until slightly heated through
- ❖ Recipe Notes: Muffins can also be eaten cold. For the quinoa, I recommend making a large batch \'7b2 cups water per each cup of dry, rinsed quinoa\'7d and saving the extra for leftovers.

Nutrition: Calories:1Total Carbohydrates: 5g;Total Fat: 7g;Protein: 6g

7) GREEK YOGURT BLUEBERRY PANCAKES

Cooking Time: 15 Minutes   **Servings:** 6

Ingredients:
- ✓ 1 1/4 cup all-purpose flour
- ✓ 2 tsp baking powder
- ✓ 1 tsp baking soda
- ✓ 1/4 tsp salt
- ✓ 1/4 cup sugar
- ✓ 3 eggs
- ✓ 3 tbsp vegan butter unsalted, melted
- ✓ 1/2 cup milk
- ✓ 1 1/2 cups Greek yogurt plain, non-fat
- ✓ 1/2 cup blueberries optional
- ✓ Toppings:
- ✓ Greek yogurt
- ✓ Mixed berries – blueberries, raspberries and blackberries

Directions:
- ❖ In a large bowl, whisk together the flour, salt, baking powder and baking soda
- ❖ In a separate bowl, whisk together butter, sugar, eggs, Greek yogurt, and milk until the mixture is smooth
- ❖ Then add in the Greek yogurt mixture from step to the dry mixture in step 1, mix to combine, allow the patter to sit for 20 minutes to get a smooth texture – if using blueberries fold them into the pancake batter
- ❖ Heat the pancake griddle, spray with non-stick butter spray or just brush with butter
- ❖ Pour the batter, in 1/4 cupful's, onto the griddle
- ❖ Cook until the bubbles on top burst and create small holes, lift up the corners of the pancake to see if they're golden browned on the bottom
- ❖ With a wide spatula, flip the pancake and cook on the other side until lightly browned
- ❖ Distribute the pancakes in among the storage containers, store in the fridge for 3 day or in the freezer for 2 months
- ❖ To Serve: Reheat microwave for 1 minute (until 80% heated through) or on the stove top, drizzle warm syrup on top, scoop of Greek yogurt, and mixed berries (including blueberries, raspberries, blackberries)

Nutrition: Calories:258;Total Carbohydrates: 33g;Total Fat: 8g;Protein: 11g

8) BREAKFAST VEGETABLE BOWL

Cooking Time: 5 Minutes   **Servings:** 2

Ingredients:
- ✓ Breakfast Bowl:
- ✓ 1 ½ cups cooked quinoa
- ✓ 1 lb asparagus[1], cut into bite-sized pieces, ends trimmed and discarded
- ✓ 1 tbsp avocado oil or olive oil
- ✓ 3 cups shredded kale leaves
- ✓ 1 batch lemony dressing
- ✓ 3 cups shredded, uncooked Brussels sprouts
- ✓ 1 avocado, peeled, pitted and thinly-sliced
- ✓ 4 eggs, cooked to your preference (optional)
- ✓ Garnishes:
- ✓ Toasted sesame seeds
- ✓ Crushed red pepper
- ✓ Sunflower seeds
- ✓ Sliced almonds
- ✓ Hummus
- ✓ Lemon Dressing:
- ✓ 2 tsp Dijon mustard
- ✓ 1 garlic clove, minced
- ✓ 2 tbsp avocado oil or olive oil
- ✓ 2 tbsp freshly-squeezed lemon juice
- ✓ Salt, to taste
- ✓ Freshly-cracked black pepper, to taste

Directions:
- ❖ In a large sauté pan over medium-high heat, add the oil
- ❖ Once heated, add the asparagus and sauté for 4-5 minutes, stirring occasionally, until tender. Remove from heat and set side
- ❖ Add the Brussels sprouts, quinoa, and cooked asparagus, and toss until combined
- ❖ Distribute among the container, store in fridge for 2-3 days
- ❖ To serve: In a large, mixing bowl combine the kale and lemony dressing. Use your fingers to massage the dressing into the kale for 2-3 minutes, or until the leaves are dark and softened, set aside. In a small mixing bowl, combine the avocado, lemon juice, dijon mustard, garlic clove, salt, and pepper. Assemble the bowls by smearing a spoonful of hummus along the side of each bowl, then portion the kale salad evenly between the four bowls. Top with the avocado slices, egg, and your desired garnishes
- ❖ Recipe Note: Feel free to sub the asparagus with your favorite vegetable(s), sautéing or roasting them until cooked

Nutrition: Calories:632;Carbs: 52g;Total Fat: 39g;Protein: 24g

9) BREAKFAST EGG-ARTICHOKE CASSEROLE

Cooking Time: 30 To 35 Minutes   **Servings:** 8

Ingredients:

- ✓ 14 ounces artichoke hearts, if using canned remember to drain them
- ✓ 16 eggs
- ✓ 1 cup shredded cheddar cheese
- ✓ 10 ounces chopped spinach, if frozen make sure it is thawed and well-drained
- ✓ 1 clove of minced garlic
- ✓ ½ cup ricotta cheese
- ✓ ½ cup parmesan cheese
- ✓ ½ tsp crushed red pepper
- ✓ 1 tsp sea salt
- ✓ ½ tsp dried thyme
- ✓ ¼ cup onion, shaved
- ✓ ¼ cup milk

Directions:

- ❖ Grease a 9 x -inch baking pan or place a piece of parchment paper inside of it.
- ❖ Turn the temperature on your oven to 350 degrees Fahrenheit.
- ❖ Crack the eggs into a bowl and whisk them well.
- ❖ Pour in the milk and whisk the two ingredients together.
- ❖ Squeeze any excess moisture from the spinach with a paper towel.
- ❖ Toss the spinach and leafless artichoke hearts into the bowl. Stir until well combined.
- ❖ Add the cheddar cheese, minced garlic, parmesan cheese, red pepper, sea salt, thyme, and onion into the bowl. Mix until all the ingredients are fully incorporated.
- ❖ Pour the eggs into the baking pan.
- ❖ Add the ricotta cheese in even dollops before placing the casserole in the oven.
- ❖ Set your timer for 30 minutes, but watch the casserole carefully after about 20 minutes. Once the eggs stop jiggling and are cooked, remove the meal from the oven. Let the casserole cool down a bit and enjoy!

Nutrition: calories: 302, fats: 18 grams, carbohydrates: grams, protein: 22 grams.

10) CAULIFLOWER RICE BOWL BREAKFAST

Cooking Time: 12 Minutes   **Servings:** 6

Ingredients:

- ✓ 1 cup cauliflower rice
- ✓ 1/2 tsp red pepper flakes
- ✓ 1 1/2 tsp curry powder
- ✓ 1/2 tbsp ginger, grated
- ✓ 1 cup vegetable stock
- ✓ 4 tomatoes, chopped
- ✓ 3 cups broccoli, chopped
- ✓ Pepper
- ✓ Salt

Directions:

- ❖ Spray instant pot from inside with cooking spray.
- ❖ Add all ingredients into the instant pot and stir well.
- ❖ Seal pot with lid and cook on high for 12 minutes.
- ❖ Once done, allow to release pressure naturally for 10 minutes then release remaining using quick release. Remove lid.
- ❖ Stir and serve.

Nutrition: Calories: 44;Fat: 0.8 g;Carbohydrates: 8.2 g;Sugar: 3.8 g;Protein: 2.8 g;Cholesterol: 0 mg

11) CUCUMBER-DILL SAVORY YOGURT

Cooking Time: 10 Minutes   **Servings:** 4

Ingredients:

- ✓ 2 cups low-fat (2%) plain Greek yogurt
- ✓ 4 tsp minced shallot
- ✓ 4 tsp freshly squeezed lemon juice
- ✓ ¼ cup chopped fresh dill
- ✓ 2 tsp olive oil
- ✓ ¼ tsp kosher salt
- ✓ Pinch freshly ground black pepper
- ✓ 2 cups chopped Persian cucumbers (about 4 medium cucumbers)

Directions:

- ❖ Combine the yogurt, shallot, lemon juice, dill, oil, salt, and pepper in a large bowl. Taste the mixture and add another pinch of salt if needed.
- ❖ Scoop ½ cup of yogurt into each of 4 containers. Place ½ cup of chopped cucumbers in each of 4 separate small containers or resealable sandwich bags.
- ❖ STORAGE: Store covered containers in the refrigerator for up to 5 days.

Nutrition: Total calories: 127; Total fat: 5g; Saturated fat: 2g; Sodium: 200mg; Carbohydrates: 9g; Fiber: 2g; Protein: 11g

12) SPICE CRANBERRY TEA

Cooking Time: 18 Minutes   **Servings: 2**

Ingredients:

- ✓ 1-ounce cranberries
- ✓ ½ lemon, juice, and zest
- ✓ 1 cinnamon stick
- ✓ 2 teabags
- ✓ ½ inch ginger, peeled and grated
- ✓ raw honey to taste
- ✓ 3 cups water

Directions:

- ❖ Start by adding all the Ingredients: except honey into a pot or saucepan.
- ❖ Bring to a boil and then simmer for about 115 minutes.
- ❖ Strain and serve the tea.
- ❖ Add honey or any other sweetener of your preference.
- ❖ Enjoy.

Nutrition: Calories: 38, Total Fat: 0.3g, Saturated Fat: 0.1, Cholesterol: 0 mg, Sodium: 2 mg, Total Carbohydrate: 10 g, Dietary Fiber: 4.9 g, Total Sugars: 1.1 g, Protein: 0.7 g, Vitamin D: 0 mcg, Calcium: 77 mg, Iron: 1 mg, Potassium: 110 mg

13) ZUCCHINI PUDDING

Cooking Time: 10 Minutes   **Servings: 4**

Ingredients:

- ✓ 2 cups zucchini, grated
- ✓ 1/2 tsp ground cardamom
- ✓ 1/4 cup swerve
- ✓ 5 oz half and half
- ✓ 5 oz unsweetened almond milk
- ✓ Pinch of salt

Directions:

- ❖ Spray instant pot from inside with cooking spray.
- ❖ Add all ingredients into the instant pot and stir well.
- ❖ Seal pot with lid and cook on high for 10 minutes.
- ❖ Once done, allow to release pressure naturally for 10 minutes then release remaining using quick release. Remove lid.
- ❖ Stir well and serve.

Nutrition: Calories: ;Fat: 4.7 g;Carbohydrates: 18.9 g;Sugar: 16 g;Protein: 1.9 g;Cholesterol: 13 mg

14) MEDITERRANEAN-STYLE BREAKFAST BURRITO

Cooking Time: 20 Minutes   **Servings: 6**

Ingredients:

- ✓ 9 eggs
- ✓ 3 tbsp chopped sun-dried tomatoes
- ✓ 6 tortillas that are 10 inches
- ✓ 2 cups baby spinach
- ✓ ½ cup feta cheese
- ✓ ¾ cups of canned refried beans
- ✓ 3 tbsp sliced black olives
- ✓ Salsa, sour cream, or any other toppings you desire

Directions:

- ❖ Wash and dry your spinach.
- ❖ Grease a medium frying pan with oil or nonstick cooking spray.
- ❖ Add the eggs into the pan and cook for about 5 minutes. Make sure you stir the eggs well, so they become scrambled.
- ❖ Combine the black olives, spinach, and sun-dried tomatoes with the eggs. Stir until the ingredients are fully incorporated.
- ❖ Add the feta cheese and then set the lid on the pan so the cheese will melt quickly.
- ❖ Spoon a bit of egg mixture into the tortilla.
- ❖ Wrap the tortillas tightly.
- ❖ Wash your pan or get a new skillet. Remember to grease the pan.
- ❖ Set each tortilla into the pan and cook each side for a couple of minutes. Once they are lightly brown, remove them from the pan and allow the burritos to cool on a serving plate. Top with your favorite condiments and enjoy!
- ❖ To store the burritos, wrap them in aluminum foil and place them in the fridge. They can be stored for up to two days.

Nutrition: calories: 252, fats: grams, carbohydrates: 21 grams, protein: 14 grams

15) DRY FRUIT HEALTHY PORRIDGE

Cooking Time: 8 Hours   **Servings:** 6

Ingredients:
- ✓ 2 cups steel-cut oats
- ✓ 1/8 tsp ground nutmeg
- ✓ 1 tsp vanilla
- ✓ 1 1/2 tsp cinnamon
- ✓ 1/2 cup dry apricots, chopped

- ✓ 1/2 cup dry cranberries, chopped
- ✓ 1/2 cup dates, chopped
- ✓ 1/2 cup raisins
- ✓ 8 cups of water
- ✓ Pinch of salt

Directions:
- ❖ Spray instant pot from inside with cooking spray.
- ❖ Add all ingredients into the instant pot and stir well.
- ❖ Seal the pot with a lid and select slow cook mode and cook on low for 8 hours.
- ❖ Stir well and serve.

Nutrition: Calories: 196;Fat: 2 g;Carbohydrates: 42 g;Sugar: 18.4 g;Protein: 4.g;Cholesterol: 0 mg

16) SCRAMBLED EGGS PESTO

Cooking Time: 10 Minutes   **Servings:** 2

Ingredients:
- ✓ 5 eggs
- ✓ 2 tbsp butter
- ✓ 2 tbsp pesto

- ✓ 4 tbsp milk
- ✓ salt to taste
- ✓ pepper to taste

Directions:
- ❖ Beat the eggs into a bowl and add salt and pepper as per your taste.
- ❖ Then, heat a pan and add the butter, then the eggs, stirring continuously.
- ❖ While stirring continuously, add the pesto.
- ❖ Switch off the heat and quickly add the creamed milk and mix it well with eggs.
- ❖ Serve hot.

Nutrition: Calories: 342, Total Fat: 29.8g, Saturated Fat: 12.3, Cholesterol: 44mg, Sodium: 345 mg, Total Carbohydrate: 3.4g, Dietary Fiber: 0.3 g, Total Sugars: 3.2 g, Protein: 16.8 g, Vitamin D: 47 mcg, Calcium: 148 mg, Iron: 2 mg, Potassium: 168 mg

17) SWEET POTATOES AND SPICED MAPLE YOGURT WITH WALNUTS BREAKFAST

Cooking Time: 45 Minutes   **Servings:** 4

Ingredients:
- ✓ 4 red garnet sweet potatoes, about 6 inches long and 2 inches in diameter
- ✓ 2 cups low-fat (2%) plain Greek yogurt

- ✓ ¼ tsp pumpkin pie spice
- ✓ 1 tbsp pure maple syrup
- ✓ ½ cup walnut pieces

Directions:
- ❖ Preheat the oven to 425°F. Line a sheet pan with a silicone baking mat or parchment paper.
- ❖ Prick the sweet potatoes in multiple places with a fork and place on the sheet pan. Bake until tender when pricked with a paring knife, 40 to 45 minutes.
- ❖ While the potatoes are baking, mix the yogurt, pumpkin pie spice, and maple syrup until well combined in a medium bowl.
- ❖ When the potatoes are cool, slice the skin down the middle vertically to open up each potato. If you'd like to eat the sweet potatoes warm, place 1 potato in each of containers and ½ cup of spiced yogurt plus 2 tbsp of walnut pieces in each of 4 other containers. If you want to eat the potatoes cold, place ½ cup of yogurt and 2 tbsp of walnuts directly on top of each of the 4 potatoes in the 4 containers.
- ❖ STORAGE: Store covered containers in the refrigerator for up to days.

Nutrition: Total calories: 350; Total fat: 13g; Saturated fat: 3g; Sodium: 72mg; Carbohydrates: 4; Fiber: 5g; Protein: 16g

18) BLUEBERRY PEACH OATMEAL

Cooking Time: 4 Hours   **Servings:** 4

Ingredients:
- ✓ 1 cup steel-cut oats
- ✓ 1/2 cup blueberries

- ✓ 3 1/2 cups unsweetened almond milk
- ✓ 7 oz can peach
- ✓ Pinch of salt

Directions:
- ❖ Spray instant pot from inside with cooking spray.
- ❖ Add all ingredients into the instant pot and stir well.
- ❖ Seal the pot with a lid and select slow cook mode and cook on low for 4 hours.
- ❖ Stir well and serve.

Nutrition: 1;Fat: 4.5 g;Carbohydrates: 25.4 g;Sugar: 8.6 g;Protein: 3.9 g;Cholesterol: 0 mg

19) MEDITERRANEAN-STYLE VEGGIE QUICHE

Cooking Time: 55 Minutes   **Servings: 8**

Ingredients:

- ✓ 1/2 cup sundried tomatoes - dry or in olive oil*
- ✓ Boiling water
- ✓ 1 prepared pie crust
- ✓ 2 tbsp vegan butter
- ✓ 1 onion, diced
- ✓ 2 cloves garlic, minced
- ✓ 1 red pepper, diced
- ✓ 1/4 cup sliced Kalamata olives
- ✓ 1 tsp dried oregano
- ✓ 1 tsp dried parsley
- ✓ 1/3 cup crumbled feta cheese
- ✓ 4 large eggs
- ✓ 1 1/4 cup milk
- ✓ 2 cups fresh spinach or 1/2 cup frozen spinach, thawed and squeezed dry
- ✓ Salt, to taste
- ✓ Pepper, to taste
- ✓ 1 cup shredded cheddar cheese, divided

Directions:

- ❖ If you're using dry sundried tomatoes - In a measure cup, add the sundried tomatoes and pour the boiling water over until just covered, allow to sit for 5 minutes or until the tomatoes are soft. The drain and chop tomatoes, set aside
- ❖ Preheat oven to 375 degrees F
- ❖ Fit a 9-inch pie plate with the prepared pie crust, then flute edges, and set aside
- ❖ In a skillet over medium high heat, melt the butter
- ❖ Add in the onion and garlic, and cook until fragrant and tender, about 3 minutes
- ❖ Add in the red pepper, cook for an additional 3 minutes, or until the peppers are just tender
- ❖ Add in the spinach, olives, oregano, and parsley, cook until the spinach is wilted (if you're using fresh) or heated through (if you're using frozen), about 5 minutes
- ❖ Remove the pan from heat, stir in the feta cheese and tomatoes, spoon the mixture into the prepared pie crust, spreading out evenly, set aside
- ❖ In a medium-sized mixing bowl, whisk together the eggs, 1/2 cup of the cheddar cheese, milk, salt, and pepper
- ❖ Pour this egg and cheese mixture evenly over the spinach mixture in the pie crust
- ❖ Sprinkle top with the remaining cheddar cheese
- ❖ Bake for 50-55 minutes, or until the crust is golden brown and the egg is set
- ❖ Allow to cool completely before slicing
- ❖ Wrap the slices in plastic wrap and then aluminum foil and place in the freezer.
- ❖ To Serve: Remove the aluminum foil and plastic wrap, and microwave for 2 minutes, then allow to rest for 30 seconds, enjoy!
- ❖ Recipe Notes: You'll find two types of sundried tomatoes available in your local grocery store—dry ones and ones packed in olive oil. Both will work for this recipe.
- ❖ If you decide to use dry ones, follow the directions in the recipe to reconstitute them. If you're using oil-packed sundried tomatoes, skip the first step and just remove them from the oil, chop them, and continue with the recipe.
- ❖ Season carefully! Between the feta, cheddar, and olives, this recipe is naturally salty.

Nutrition: Calories:239;Carbs: ;Total Fat: 15g;Protein: 7g

20) SCRAMBLED EGGS MEDITERRANEAN-STYLE

Cooking Time: 10 Minutes   **Servings:** 2

Ingredients:

- ✓ 1 tbsp oil
- ✓ 1 yellow pepper, diced
- ✓ 2 spring onions, sliced
- ✓ 8 cherry tomatoes, quartered
- ✓ 2 tbsp sliced black olives
- ✓ 1 tbsp capers
- ✓ 4 eggs
- ✓ 1/4 tsp dried oregano
- ✓ Black pepper
- ✓ Topping:
- ✓ Fresh parsley, to serve

Directions:

- ❖ In a frying pan over medium heat, add the oil
- ❖ Once heated, add the diced pepper and chopped spring onions, cook for a few minutes, until slightly soft
- ❖ Add in the quartered tomatoes, olives and capers, and cook for 1 more minute
- ❖ Crack the eggs into the pan, immediately scramble with a spoon or spatula
- ❖ Sprinkle with oregano and plenty of black pepper, and stir until the eggs are fully cooked
- ❖ Distribute the eggs evenly into the containers, store in the fridge for 2-3 days
- ❖ To Serve: Reheat in the microwave for 30 seconds or in a toaster oven until warmed through

Nutrition: Calories:249;Carbs: 13g;Total Fat: 17g;Protein: 14g

21) PUDDING WITH CHIA

Cooking Time: 15 Minutes   **Servings:** 2

Ingredients:

- ✓ ½ cup chia seeds
- ✓ 2 cups milk
- ✓ 1 tbsp honey

Directions:

- ❖ Combine and mix the chia seeds, milk, and honey in a bowl.
- ❖ Put the mixture in the freezer and let it set.
- ❖ Take the pudding out of the freezer only when you see that the pudding has thickened.
- ❖ Serve chilled.

Nutrition: Calories: 429, Total Fat: 22.4g, Saturated Fat: 4.9, Cholesterol: 20 mg, Sodium: 124 mg, Total Carbohydrate: 44.g, Dietary Fiber: 19.5 g, Total Sugars: 19.6 g, Protein: 17.4 g, Vitamin D: 1 mcg, Calcium: 648 mg, Iron: 4 mg, Potassium: 376 mg

22) RICE BOWLS FOR BREAKFAST

Cooking Time: 8 Minutes   **Servings:** 4

Ingredients:

- ✓ 1 cup of brown rice
- ✓ 1 tsp ground cinnamon
- ✓ 1/4 cup almonds, sliced
- ✓ 2 tbsp sunflower seeds
- ✓ 1/4 cup pecans, chopped
- ✓ 1/4 cup walnuts, chopped
- ✓ 2 cup unsweetened almond milk
- ✓ Pinch of salt

Directions:

- ❖ Spray instant pot from inside with cooking spray.
- ❖ Add all ingredients into the instant pot and stir well.
- ❖ Seal pot with lid and cook on high for 8 minutes.
- ❖ Once done, allow to release pressure naturally for 5 minutes then release remaining using quick release. Remove lid.
- ❖ Stir well and serve.

Nutrition: Calories: 291;Fat: 12 g;Carbohydrates: 40.1 g;Sugar: 0.4 g;Protein: 7.g;Cholesterol: 0 mg

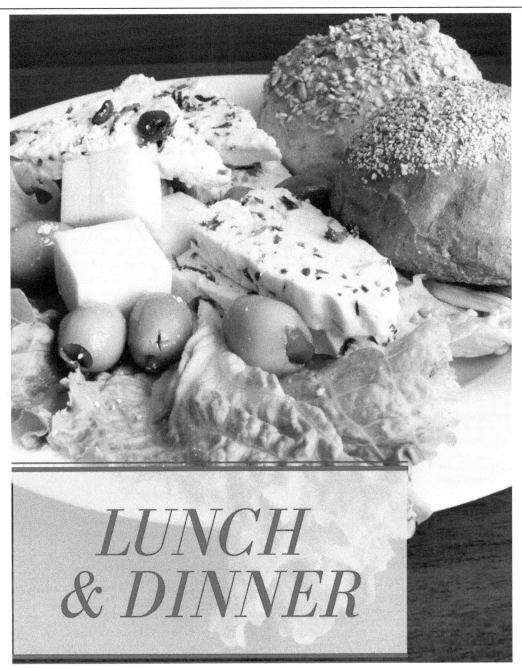

LUNCH & DINNER

23) MEDITERRANEAN-STYLE PEARL COUSCOUS

Cooking Time: 10 Minutes   **Servings: 6**

Ingredients:
- ✓ For the Lemon Dill Vinaigrette:
- ✓ 1 large lemon, juice of
- ✓ 1/3 cup Extra virgin olive oil
- ✓ 1 tsp dill weed
- ✓ 1 tsp garlic powder
- ✓ Salt and pepper
- ✓ For the Israeli Couscous:
- ✓ 2 cups Pearl Couscous, Israeli Couscous
- ✓ Extra virgin olive oil
- ✓ 2 cups grape tomatoes, halved
- ✓ 1/3 cup finely chopped red onions
- ✓ 1/2 English cucumber, finely chopped
- ✓ 15 oz can chickpeas
- ✓ 14 oz can good quality artichoke hearts, roughly chopped if needed
- ✓ 1/2 cup good pitted kalamata olives
- ✓ 15–20 fresh basil leaves, roughly chopped or torn; more for garnish
- ✓ 3 oz fresh baby mozzarella or feta cheese, optional
- ✓ Water

Directions:
- ❖ Make the lemon-dill vinaigrette, place the lemon juice, olive oil, dill weed, garlic powder, salt and pepper in a bowl, whisk together to combine and set aside
- ❖ In a medium-sized heavy pot, heat two tbsp of olive oil
- ❖ Sauté the couscous in the olive oil briefly until golden brown, then add cups of boiling water (or follow the instructed on the package), and cook according to package.
- ❖ Once done, drain in a colander, set aside in a bowl and allow to cool
- ❖ In a large mixing bowl, combine the extra virgin olive oil, grape tomatoes, red onions, cucumber, chickpeas, artichoke hearts, and kalamata olives
- ❖ Then add in the couscous and the basil, mix together gently
- ❖ Now, give the lemon-dill vinaigrette a quick whisk and add to the couscous salad, mix to combine
- ❖ Taste and adjust salt, if needed
- ❖ Distribute among the containers, store for 2-3 days
- ❖ To Serve: Add in the mozzarella cheese, garnish with more fresh basil and enjoy

Nutrition: Calories:393;Carbs: 57g;Total Fat: 13g;Protein: 13g

24) POTATO WITH TUNA SALAD

Cooking Time: Nil   **Servings: 4**

Ingredients:
- ✓ 1-pound baby potatoes, scrubbed, boiled
- ✓ 1 cup tuna chunks, drained
- ✓ 1 cup cherry tomatoes, halved
- ✓ 1 cup medium onion, thinly sliced
- ✓ 8 pitted black olives
- ✓ 2 medium hard-boiled eggs, sliced
- ✓ 1 head Romaine lettuce
- ✓ Honey lemon mustard dressing
- ✓ ¼ cup olive oil
- ✓ 2 tbsp lemon juice
- ✓ 1 tbsp Dijon mustard
- ✓ 1 tsp dill weed, chopped
- ✓ Salt as needed
- ✓ Pepper as needed

Directions:
- ❖ Take a small glass bowl and mix in your olive oil, honey, lemon juice, Dijon mustard and dill
- ❖ Season the mix with pepper and salt
- ❖ Add in the tuna, baby potatoes, cherry tomatoes, red onion, green beans, black olives and toss everything nicely
- ❖ Arrange your lettuce leaves on a beautiful serving dish to make the base of your salad
- ❖ Top them up with your salad mixture and place the egg slices
- ❖ Drizzle it with the previously prepared Salad Dressing
- ❖ Serve hot
- ❖ Meal Prep/Storage Options: Store in airtight containers in your fridge for 1-2 days. Keep the fish and salad ingredients separated, mix together before serving!

Nutrition: Calories: 406;Fat: 22g;Carbohydrates: 28g;Protein: 26g

25) MEDITERRANEAN-STYLE PASTA SALAD

Cooking Time: 25 Minutes **Servings: 8**

Ingredients:
- ✓ Salad:
- ✓ 8 oz pasta, I used farfalle, any smallish pasta works great!
- ✓ 1 cup rotisserie chicken, chopped
- ✓ 1/2 cup sun-dried tomatoes packed in oil, drained and coarsely chopped
- ✓ 1/2 cup jarred marinated artichoke hearts, drained and coarsely chopped
- ✓ 1/2 of 1 full English cucumber, chopped
- ✓ 1/3 cup kalamata olives, coarsely chopped
- ✓ 2 cups lightly packed fresh arugula
- ✓ 1/4 cup fresh flat leaf Italian parsley, coarsely chopped
- ✓ 1 small avocado, pit removed and coarsely chopped
- ✓ 1/3 cup feta cheese

- ✓ Dressing:
- ✓ 4 tbsp red wine vinegar
- ✓ 1 ½ tbsp
- ✓ dijon mustard, do not use regular mustard
- ✓ 1/2 tsp dried oregano
- ✓ 1 tsp dried basil
- ✓ 1 clove garlic, minced
- ✓ 1-2 tsp honey
- ✓ 1/2 cup olive oil
- ✓ 3 tbsp freshly squeezed lemon juice
- ✓ Fine sea salt, to taste
- ✓ Freshly cracked pepper, to taste

Directions:
- ❖ Prepare the pasta according to package directions until al dente, drain the pasta and allow it to completely cool to room temperature, then add it to a large bowl
- ❖ Add in the chopped rotisserie chicken, chopped cucumber, coarsely chopped kalamata olives, coarsely chopped sun-dried tomatoes, coarsely chopped artichoke hearts, arugula, and parsley, toss
- ❖ Distribute the salad among the containers, store for 2-days
- ❖ Prepare the dressing - In a mason jar with a lid, combine the red wine vinegar, Dijon mustard, garlic, 1/2 tsp salt (or to taste), dried oregano, dried basil and 1/tsp pepper (or to taste, honey (add to sweetness preference), olive oil, and freshly squeezed lemon juice, place the lid on the mason jar and shake to combine, store in fridge
- ❖ To Serve: Add in the avocado and feta cheese to the salad, drizzle with the dressing, adjust any seasonings salt and pepper to taste, serve

Nutrition: Calories:32Carbs: 24g;Total Fat: 21g;Protein: 8g

26) AVOCADO LEMON HERB CHICKEN SALAD

Cooking Time: 15 Minutes **Servings: 4**

Ingredients:
- ✓ Marinade/ Dressing:
- ✓ 2 tbsp olive oil
- ✓ 1/4 cup fresh lemon juice
- ✓ 2 tbsp water
- ✓ 2 tbsp fresh chopped parsley
- ✓ 2 tsp garlic, minced
- ✓ 1 tsp each dried thyme and dried rosemary
- ✓ 1 tsp salt
- ✓ 1/4 tsp cracked pepper, or to taste

- ✓ 1 pound skinless & boneless chicken thigh fillets or chicken breasts
- ✓ Salad:
- ✓ 4 cups Romaine lettuce leaves, washed and dried
- ✓ 1 large avocado, pitted, peeled and sliced
- ✓ 8 oz feta cheese
- ✓ 1 cup grape tomatoes, halved
- ✓ 1/4 of a red onion, sliced, optional
- ✓ 1/4 cup diced bacon, trimmed of rind and fat (optional)
- ✓ Lemon wedges, to serve

Directions:
- ❖ In a large jug, whisk together the olive oil, lemon juice, water, chopped parsley, garlic, thyme, rosemary, salt, and pepper
- ❖ Pour half of the marinade into a large, shallow dish and refrigerate the remaining marinade to use as the dressing
- ❖ Add the chicken to the marinade in the bowl, allow the chicken to marinade for 15- minutes (or up to two hours in the refrigerator if you can)
- ❖ In the meantime,
- ❖ Once the chicken is ready, place a skillet or grill over medium-high heat add 1 tbsp of oil in, sear the chicken on both sides until browned and cooked through about 7 minutes per side, depending on thickness, and discard of the marinade
- ❖ Allow the chicken to rest for 5 minutes, slice and then allow the chicken to cool
- ❖ Distribute among the containers, and keep in the refrigerator
- ❖ To Serve: Reheat the chicken in the microwave for 30 seconds to 1 minutes. In a bowl, add the romaine lettuce, avocado, feta cheese, grape tomatoes, red onion and bacon, mix to combine. Arrange the chicken over salad. Drizzle the salad with the Untouched dressing. Serve with lemon wedges and enjoy!

Nutrition: Calories:378;Carbs: 6g;Total Fat: 22g;Protein: 31g

27) LEEKS, GREENS, AND POTATOES IN GREEK-STYLE BRAISED PORK

Cooking Time: 1 Hour 40 Minutes   **Servings:** 4

Ingredients:

- ✓ 1 tbsp olive oil, plus 2 tsp
- ✓ 1¼ pounds boneless pork loin chops, fat cap removed and cut into 1-inch pieces
- ✓ 2 leeks, white and light green parts quartered vertically and thinly sliced
- ✓ 1 bulb fennel, quartered and thinly sliced
- ✓ 1 cup chopped onion
- ✓ 1 tsp chopped garlic
- ✓ 2 cups reduced-sodium chicken broth
- ✓ 1 tsp fennel seed
- ✓ 1 tsp dried oregano
- ✓ ½ tsp kosher salt
- ✓ 1 pound baby red potatoes, halved
- ✓ 1 bunch chard, including stems, chopped
- ✓ 2 tbsp freshly squeezed lemon juice

Directions:

- ❖ Heat tbsp of oil in a soup pot or Dutch oven over medium-high heat. When the oil is shimmering, add the pork cubes and brown for about 6 minutes, turning the cubes over after 3 minutes. Remove the pork to a plate.
- ❖ Add the remaining tsp of oil to the same pot and add the leeks, fennel, onion, and garlic. Cook for 3 minutes.
- ❖ Pour the broth into the pan, scraping up any browned bits on the bottom. Add the fennel seed, oregano, and salt, and add the pork, plus any juices that may have accumulated on the plate. Make sure the pork is submerged in the liquid. Place the potatoes on top, then place the chard on top of the potatoes.
- ❖ Cover, turn down the heat to low, and simmer for 1½ hours, until the pork is tender. When the pork is done cooking, add the lemon juice. Taste and add more salt if needed. Cool.
- ❖ Scoop 2 cups of the mixture into each of 4 containers.
- ❖ STORAGE: Store covered containers in the refrigerator for up to 5 days.

Nutrition: Total calories: 3; Total fat: 13g; Saturated fat: 3g; Sodium: 1,607mg; Carbohydrates: 33g; Fiber: 8g; Protein: 34g

28) DELIZIOSA BROCCOLI TORTELLINI SALAD

Cooking Time: 20 To 25 Minutes   **Servings:** 12

Ingredients:

- ✓ 1 cup sunflower seeds, or any of your favorite seeds
- ✓ 3 heads of broccoli, fresh is best!
- ✓ ½ cup sugar
- ✓ 20 ounces cheese-filled tortellini
- ✓ 1 onion
- ✓ 2 tsp cider vinegar
- ✓ ½ cup mayonnaise
- ✓ 1 cup raisins-optional

Directions:

- ❖ Cut your broccoli into florets and chop the onion.
- ❖ Follow the directions to make the cheese-filled tortellini. Once they are cooked, drain and rinse them with cold water.
- ❖ In a bowl, combine your mayonnaise, sugar, and vinegar. Whisk well to give the ingredients a dressing consistency.
- ❖ In a separate large bowl, toss in your seeds, onion, tortellini, raisins, and broccoli.
- ❖ Pour the salad dressing into the large bowl and toss the ingredients together. You will want to ensure everything is thoroughly mixed as you'll want a taste of the salad dressing with every bite!

Nutrition: calories: 272, fats: 8.1 grams, carbohydrates: 38.grams, protein: 5 grams.

29) AVOCADO ARUGULA SALAD

Cooking Time: 15 Minutes   **Servings:** 4

Ingredients:

- ✓ 4 cups packed baby arugula
- ✓ 4 green onions, tops trimmed, chopped
- ✓ 1½ cups shelled fava beans
- ✓ 3 Persian cucumbers, chopped
- ✓ 2 cups grape tomatoes, halved
- ✓ 1 jalapeno pepper, sliced
- ✓ 1 avocado, cored, peeled, and roughly chopped
- ✓ lemon juice, 1½ lemons
- ✓ ½ cup extra virgin olive oil
- ✓ salt
- ✓ pepper
- ✓ 1 garlic clove, finely chopped
- ✓ 2 tbsp fresh cilantro, finely chopped
- ✓ 2 tbsp fresh mint, finely chopped

Directions:

- ❖ Place the lemon-honey vinaigrette Ingredients: in a small bowl and whisk them well.
- ❖ In a large mixing bowl, add baby arugula, fava beans, green onions, tomatoes, cucumbers, and jalapeno.
- ❖ Divide the whole salad among four containers.
- ❖ Before serving, dress the salad with the vinaigrette and toss.
- ❖ Add the avocado to the salad.
- ❖ Enjoy!

Nutrition: Calories: 229, Total Fat: 11.1 g, Saturated Fat: 2.5 g, Cholesterol: 0 mg, Sodium: 24 mg, Total Carbohydrate: 32.1 g, Dietary Fiber: 12 g, Total Sugars: 10.1 g, Protein: 3 g, Vitamin D: 0 mcg, Calcium: 163 mg, Iron: 3 mg, Potassium: 1166 mg

30) QUINOA STUFFED EGGPLANT AND TAHINI SAUCE

Cooking Time: 30 Minutes   **Servings: 2**

Ingredients:

- ✓ 1 eggplant
- ✓ 2 tbsp olive oil, divided
- ✓ 1 medium shallot, diced, about 1/2 cup
- ✓ 1 cup chopped button mushrooms, about 2 cups whole
- ✓ 5-6 Tuttorosso whole plum tomatoes, chopped
- ✓ 1 tbsp tomato juice from the can
- ✓ 1 tbsp chopped fresh parsley, plus more to garnish
- ✓ 2 garlic cloves, minced
- ✓ 1/2 cup cooked quinoa
- ✓ 1/2 tsp ground cumin
- ✓ Salt, to taste
- ✓ Pepper, to taste
- ✓ 1 tbsp tahini
- ✓ 1 tsp lemon juice
- ✓ 1/2 tsp garlic powder
- ✓ Water to thin

Directions:

- ❖ Preheat the oven to 425 degrees F
- ❖ Prepare the eggplant by cutting it in half lengthwise and scoop out some of the flesh
- ❖ Place it on a baking sheet, drizzle with 1 tbsp of oil, sprinkle with salt
- ❖ Bake for 20 minutes
- ❖ In the meantime, add the remaining oil in a large skillet
- ❖ Once heated, add the shallots and mushrooms, sauté until mushrooms have softened, about 5 minutes Add in the tomatoes, quinoa and spices, cook until the liquid has evaporated
- ❖ Once the eggplant has cooked, reduce the oven temperature to 350 degrees F
- ❖ Stuff each half with the tomato-quinoa mixture
- ❖ Bake for another 10 minutes
- ❖ Allow to cool completely
- ❖ Distribute among the containers, store for 2 days
- ❖ To Serve: Reheat in the microwave for 1-2 minutes or until heated through. Quickly whisk together tahini, lemon, garlic, water and a sprinkle of salt and pepper, drizzle tahini over eggplants and sprinkle with parsley and enjoy.

Nutrition: Calories:345;Carbs: 38g;Total Fat: 19g;Protein: 9g

31) ITALIAN-STYLE LASAGNA

Cooking Time: 1 Hour 15 Minutes   **Servings: 8**

Ingredients:

- ✓ Lasagna noodles, oven-ready are the best, easiest, and quickest
- ✓ ⅓ cup flour
- ✓ 2 tbsp chives, divided and chopped
- ✓ ½ cup white wine
- ✓ 2 tbsp olive oil
- ✓ 1 ½ tbsp thyme
- ✓ 1 tsp salt
- ✓ 1 ¼ cups shallots, chopped
- ✓ 1 cup boiled water
- ✓ ½ cup Parmigiano-Reggiano cheese
- ✓ 3 cups milk, reduced-fat and divided
- ✓ 1 tbsp butter
- ✓ ⅓ cup cream cheese, less fat is the best choice
- ✓ 6 cloves of garlic, divided and minced
- ✓ ½ tsp ground black pepper, divided
- ✓ 4 ounces dried shiitake mushrooms, sliced
- ✓ 1 ounce dried porcini mushrooms, sliced
- ✓ 8 ounces cremini mushrooms, sliced

Directions:

- ❖ Keeping your mushrooms separated, drain them all and return them to separate containers.
- ❖ Bring 1 cup of water to a boil and cook your porcini mushrooms for a half hour.
- ❖ Preheat your oven to 0 degrees Fahrenheit.
- ❖ Set a large pan on your stove and turn the burner to medium-high heat.
- ❖ Add your butter and let it melt.
- ❖ Combine the olive oil and shallots. Stir the mixture and let it cook for 3 minutes.
- ❖ Pour half of the pepper, half of the salt, and mushrooms into the pan. Allow the mixture to cook for 6 to minutes.
- ❖ While stirring, add half of the garlic and thyme. Continue to stir for 1 minute.
- ❖ Pour the wine and turn your burner temperature to high. Let the mixture boil and watch the liquid evaporate for a couple of minutes to reduce it slightly.
- ❖ Turn off the burner and remove the pan from heat.
- ❖ Add the cream cheese and chives. Stir thoroughly.
- ❖ Set a medium-sized skillet on medium-high heat and add 1 tbsp of oil. Let the oil come to a simmer.
- ❖ Add the last of the garlic to the pan and saute for 30 seconds.
- ❖ Pour in 2 ⅓ cup milk and the liquid from the porcini mushrooms. Stir the mixture and allow it to boil.
- ❖ In a bowl, combine ¼ cup of milk and the flour. Add this mixture to the heated pan. Stir until the mixture starts to thicken.
- ❖ Grease a pan and add ½ cup of sauce along with a row of noodles.
- ❖ Spread half of the mushroom mixture on top of the noodles.
- ❖ Repeat the process, but make sure you top the lasagna with mushrooms and cheese.
- ❖ Turn your timer to 45 minutes and set the pan into the oven.
- ❖ Remember to garnish the lasagna with chives before enjoying!

Nutrition: calories: 268, fats: 12.6 grams, carbohydrates: 29 grams, protein: 10 grams.

32) TUNA AND VEGETABLE MIX

Cooking Time: 15 Minutes   **Servings:** 4

Ingredients:

- ¼ cup extra-virgin olive oil, divided
- 1 tbsp rice vinegar
- 1 tsp kosher salt, divided
- ¾ tsp Dijon mustard
- ¾ tsp honey
- 4 ounces baby gold beets, thinly sliced
- 4 ounces fennel bulb, trimmed and thinly sliced
- 4 ounces baby turnips, thinly sliced
- 6 ounces Granny Smith apple, very thinly sliced
- 2 tsp sesame seeds, toasted
- 6 ounces tuna steaks
- ½ tsp black pepper
- 1 tbsp fennel fronds, torn

Directions:

- In a large bowl, add 2 tbsp of oil, ½ a tsp of salt, honey, vinegar, and mustard.
- Give the mixture a nice mix.
- Add fennel, beets, apple, and turnips; mix and toss until everything is evenly coated.
- Sprinkle with sesame seeds and toss well.
- In a cast-iron skillet, heat 2 tbsp of oil over high heat.
- Carefully season the tuna with ½ a tsp of salt and pepper
- Place the tuna in the skillet and cook for about 3 minutes total, giving 1½ minutes per side.
- Remove the tuna and slice it up.
- Place in containers with the vegetable mix.
- Serve with the fennel mix, and enjoy!

Nutrition: Calories: 443, Total Fat: 17.1 g, Saturated Fat: 2.6 g, Cholesterol: 21 mg, Sodium: 728 mg, Total Carbohydrate: 62.5 g, Dietary Fiber: 12.3 g, Total Sugars: 45 g, Protein: 16.5 g, Vitamin D: 0 mcg, Calcium: 79 mg, Iron: 4 mg, Potassium: 1008 mg

33) SPICY BURGERS

Cooking Time: 25-30 Minutes   **Servings:** 6/2 Chops Each

Ingredients:

- Medium onion (1)
- Fresh parsley (3 tbsp.)
- Clove of garlic (1)
- Ground allspice (.75 tsp.)
- Pepper (.75 tsp.)
- Ground nutmeg (.25 tsp.)
- Cinnamon (.5 tsp.)
- Salt (.5 tsp.)
- Fresh mint (2 tbsp.)
- 90% lean ground beef (1.5 lb.)
- Optional: Cold Tzatziki sauce

Directions:

- Finely chop/mince the parsley, mint, garlic, and onions.
- Whisk the nutmeg, salt, cinnamon, pepper, allspice, garlic, mint, parsley, and onion.
- Add the beef and prepare six (6 2x4-inch oblong patties.
- Use the medium temperature setting to grill the patties or broil them four inches from the heat source for four to six minutes per side.
- When they're done, the meat thermometer will register 160° Fahrenheit. Serve with the sauce if desired.

Nutrition: Calories: 231;Protein: 32 grams;Fat: 9 grams

34) TUNA BOWL AND KALE

Cooking Time: 15 To 20 Minutes   **Servings:** 6

Ingredients:

- 3 tbsp extra virgin olive oil
- 1 ½ tsp minced garlic
- ¼ cup of capers
- 2 tsp sugar
- 15 ounce can of drained and rinsed great northern beans
- 1 pound chopped kale with the center ribs removed
- ½ tsp ground black pepper
- 1 cup chopped onion
- 2 ½ ounces of drained sliced olives
- ¼ tsp sea salt
- ¼ tsp crushed red pepper
- 6 ounces of tuna in olive oil, do not drain

Directions:

- Place a large pot, like a stockpot, on your stove and turn the burner to high heat.
- Fill the pot about 3-quarters of the way full with water and let it come to a boil.
- Add the kale and cook for 2 minutes.
- Drain the kale and set it aside.
- Turn the heat down to medium and place the empty pot back on the burner.
- Add the oil and onion. Saute for 3 to 4 minutes.
- Combine the garlic into the oil mixture and saute for another minute.
- Add the capers, olives, and red pepper.
- Cook the ingredients for another minute while stirring.
- Pour in the sugar and stir while you toss in the kale. Mix all the ingredients thoroughly and ensure the kale is thoroughly coated.
- Cover the pot and set the timer for 8 minutes.
- Turn off the heat and add in the tuna, pepper, beans, salt, and any other herbs that will make this one of the best Mediterranean-Style dishes you've ever made.

Nutrition: calories: 265, fats: 12 grams, carbohydrates: 26 grams, protein: 16 grams.

35) POMODORO SOUP

Cooking Time: 30 Minutes　　　　**Servings: 8**

Ingredients:
- ✓ 4 tbsp olive oil
- ✓ 2 medium yellow onions, thinly sliced
- ✓ 1 tsp salt (extra for taste if needed)
- ✓ 2 tsp curry powder
- ✓ 1 tsp red curry powder
- ✓ 1 tsp ground coriander
- ✓ 1 tsp ground cumin
- ✓ ¼-½ tsp red pepper flakes
- ✓ 1 15-ounce can diced tomatoes, undrained
- ✓ 1 28-ounce can diced or plum tomatoes, undrained
- ✓ 5½ cups water (vegetable broth or chicken broth also usable)
- ✓ 1 14-ounce can coconut milk
- ✓ optional add-ins: cooked brown rice, lemon wedges, fresh thyme, etc.

Directions:
- ❖ Heat oil in a medium-sized pot over medium heat.
- ❖ Add onions and salt and cook for about 10-1minutes until browned.
- ❖ Stir in curry powder, coriander, red pepper flakes, cumin, and cook for seconds, being sure to keep stirring well.
- ❖ Add tomatoes and water (or broth if you prefer).
- ❖ Simmer the mixture for 1minutes.
- ❖ Take an immersion blender and puree the mixture until a soupy consistency is achieved.
- ❖ Enjoy as it is, or add some extra add-ins for a more flavorful experience

Nutrition: Calories: 217, Total Fat: 19.3 g, Saturated Fat: 11.5 g, Cholesterol: 0 mg, Sodium: 40 mg, Total Carbohydrate: 12.1 g, Dietary Fiber: 3.g, Total Sugars: 7.1 g, Protein: 3 g, Vitamin D: 0 mcg, Calcium: 58 mg, Iron: 2 mg, Potassium: 570 mg

36) ONION CHEESE SOUP

Cooking Time: 25 Minutes　　　　**Servings: 4**

Ingredients:
- ✓ 2 large onions, finely sliced
- ✓ 2 cups vegetable stock
- ✓ 1 tsp brown sugar
- ✓ 1 cup red wine
- ✓ 1 measure of brandy
- ✓ 1 tsp herbs de Provence
- ✓ 4 slices stale bread
- ✓ 4 ounces grated strong cheese
- ✓ 1-ounce grated parmesan
- ✓ 1 tbsp plain flour
- ✓ 2 tbsp olive oil
- ✓ 1-ounce butter
- ✓ salt
- ✓ pepper

Directions:
- ❖ Heat oil and butter in a pan over medium-high heat.
- ❖ Add onions and brown sugar.
- ❖ Cook until the onions are golden brown.
- ❖ Pour brandy and flambé, making sure to keep stirring until the flames are out.
- ❖ Add plain flour and herbs de Provence and keep stirring well.
- ❖ Slowly add the stock and red wine.
- ❖ Season well and simmer for 20 minutes, making sure to add water if the soup becomes too thick.
- ❖ Ladle the soup into jars.
- ❖ Before serving, place rounds of stale bread on top.
- ❖ Add strong cheese.
- ❖ Garnish with some parmesan.
- ❖ Place the bowls under a hot grill or in an oven until the cheese has melted.

Nutrition: Calories: 403, Total Fat: 22.4 g, Saturated Fat: 10.9 g, Cholesterol: 41 mg, Sodium: 886 mg, Total Carbohydrate: 24.9 g, Dietary Fiber: 3.6 g, Total Sugars: 7 g, Protein: 16.2 g, Vitamin D: 4 mcg, Calcium: 371 mg, Iron: 1 mg, Potassium: 242 mg

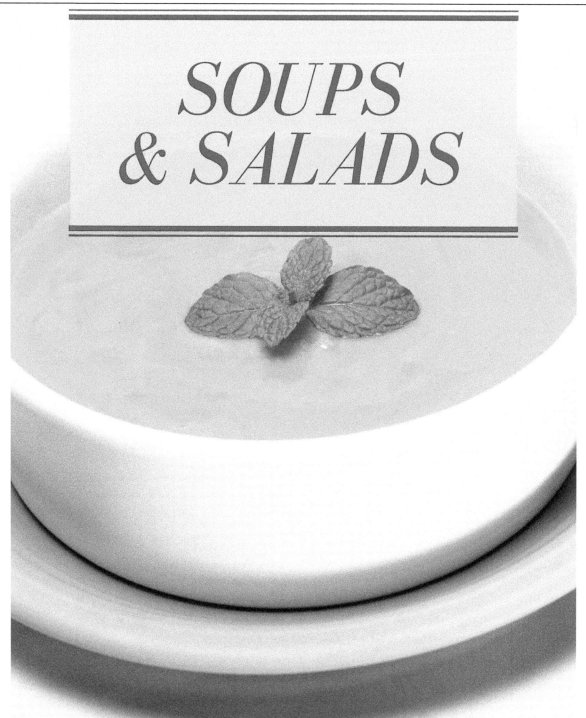

SOUPS & SALADS

37) TURKEY MEATBALL WITH DITALINI SOUP

Cooking Time: 40 Minutes   **Servings:** 4

Ingredients:

- meatballs:
- 1 pound 93% lean ground turkey
- 1/3 cup seasoned breadcrumbs
- 3 tbsp grated Pecorino Romano cheese
- 1 large egg, beaten
- 1 clove crushed garlic
- 1 tbsp fresh minced parsley
- 1/2 tsp kosher salt
- Soup:
- cooking spray
- 1 tsp olive oil
- 1/2 cup chopped onion
- 1/2 cup chopped celery
- 1/2 cup chopped carrot
- 3 cloves minced garlic
- 1 can (28 ounces diced San Marzano tomatoes
- 4 cups reduced sodium chicken broth
- 4 torn basil leaves
- 2 bay leaves
- 1 cup ditalini pasta
- 1 cup zucchini, diced small
- Parmesan rind, optional
- Grated parmesan cheese, optional for serving

Directions:

- ❖ Thoroughly combine turkey with egg, garlic, parsley, salt, pecorino and breadcrumbs in a bowl.
- ❖ Make 30 equal sized meatballs out of this mixture.
- ❖ Preheat olive oil in the insert of the Instant Pot on Sauté mode.
- ❖ Sear the meatballs in the heated oil in batches, until brown.
- ❖ Set the meatballs aside in a plate.
- ❖ Add more oil to the insert of the Instant Pot.
- ❖ Stir in carrots, garlic, celery, and onion. Sauté for 4 minutes.
- ❖ Add basil, bay leaves, tomatoes, and Parmesan rind.
- ❖ Return the seared meatballs to the pot along with the broth.
- ❖ Secure and sear the Instant Pot lid and select Manual mode for 15 minutes at high pressure.
- ❖ Once done, release the pressure completely then remove the lid.
- ❖ Add zucchini and pasta, cook it for 4 minutes on Sauté mode.
- ❖ Garnish with cheese and basil.
- ❖ Serve.

Nutrition: Calories: 261;Carbohydrate: 11.2g;Protein: 36.6g;Fat: 7g;Sugar: 3g;Sodium: 198g

38) LOVELY MINT AVOCADO CHILLED SOUP

Cooking Time: 5 Minutes   **Servings:** 2

Ingredients:

- 1 cup coconut milk, chilled
- 1 medium ripe avocado
- 1 tbsp lime juice
- Salt, to taste
- 20 fresh mint leaves

Directions:

- ❖ Put all the ingredients into an immersion blender and blend until a thick mixture is formed.
- ❖ Allow to cool in the fridge for about 10 minutes and serve chilled.

Nutrition: Calories: 286;Carbs: 12.6g;Fats: 26.9g;Proteins: 4.2g;Sodium: 70mg;Sugar: 4.6g

39) CLASSIC SPLIT PEA SOUP

Cooking Time: 30 Minutes   **Servings:** 6

Ingredients:

- 3 tbsp butter
- 1 onion diced
- 2 ribs celery diced
- 2 carrots diced
- 6 oz. diced ham
- 1 lb. dry split peas sorted and rinsed
- 6 cups chicken stock
- 2 bay leaves
- kosher salt and black pepper

Directions:

- ❖ Set your Instant Pot on Sauté mode and melt butter in it.
- ❖ Stir in celery, onion, carrots, salt, and pepper.
- ❖ Sauté them for 5 minutes then stir in split peas, ham bone, chicken stock, and bay leaves.
- ❖ Seal and lock the Instant Pot lid then select Manual mode for 15 minutes at high pressure.
- ❖ Once done, release the pressure completely then remove the lid.
- ❖ Remove the ham bone and separate meat from the bone.
- ❖ Shred or dice the meat and return it to the soup.
- ❖ Adjust seasoning as needed then serve warm.
- ❖ Enjoy.

Nutrition: Calories: 190;Carbohydrate: 30.5g;Protein: 8g;Fat: 3.5g;Sugar: 4.2g;Sodium: 461mg

40) SPECIAL BUTTERNUT SQUASH SOUP

Cooking Time: 40 Minutes **Servings: 4**

Ingredients:
- 1 tbsp olive oil
- 1 medium yellow onion chopped
- 1 large carrot chopped
- 1 celery rib chopped
- 3 cloves of garlic minced
- 2 lbs. butternut squash, peeled chopped
- 2 cups vegetable broth
- 1 green apple peeled, cored, and chopped
- 1/4 tsp ground cinnamon
- 1 sprig fresh thyme
- 1 sprig fresh rosemary
- 1 tsp kosher salt
- 1/2 tsp black pepper
- Pinch of nutmeg optional

Directions:
- Preheat olive oil in the insert of the Instant Pot on Sauté mode.
- Add celery, carrots, and garlic, sauté for 5 minutes.
- Stir in squash, broth, cinnamon, apple nutmeg, rosemary, thyme, salt, and pepper.
- Mix well gently then seal and secure the lid.
- Select Manual mode to cook for 10 minutes at high pressure.
- Once done, release the pressure completely then remove the lid.
- Puree the soup using an immersion blender.
- Serve warm.

Nutrition: Calories: 282;Carbohydrate: 50g;Protein: 13g;Fat: 4.7g;Sugar: 12.8g;Sodium: 213mg

41) LOVELY CREAMY CILANTRO LIME COLESLAW

Cooking Time: 10 Minutes **Servings: 2**

Ingredients:
- ¾ avocado
- 1 lime, juiced
- 1/8 cup water
- Cilantro, to garnish
- 6 oz coleslaw, bagged
- 1/8 cup cilantro leaves
- 1 garlic clove
- ¼ tsp salt

Directions:
- Put garlic and cilantro in a food processor and process until chopped.
- Add lime juice, avocado and water and pulse until creamy.
- Put coleslaw in a large bowl and stir in the avocado mixture.
- Refrigerate for a few hours before serving.

Nutrition: Calories: 240;Carbs: 17.4g;Fats: 19.6g;Proteins: 2.8g;Sodium: 0mg;Sugar: 0.5g

42) CLASSIC SNAP PEA SALAD

Cooking Time: 15 Minutes **Servings: 2**

Ingredients:
- 1/8 cup lemon juice
- ½ clove garlic, crushed
- 4 ounces cauliflower riced
- 1/8 cup olive oil
- ¼ tsp coarse grain Dijon mustard
- ½ tsp granulated stevia
- ¼ cup sugar snap peas, ends removed and each pod cut into three pieces
- 1/8 cup chives
- 1/8 cup red onions, minced Sea salt and black pepper, to taste
- ¼ cup almonds, sliced

Directions:
- Pour water in a pot fitted with a steamer basket and bring water to a boil.
- Place riced cauliflower in the steamer basket and season with sea salt.
- Cover the pot and steam for about 10 minutes until tender.
- Drain the cauliflower and dish out in a bowl to refrigerate for about 1 hour.
- Meanwhile, make a dressing by mixing olive oil, lemon juice, garlic, mustard, stevia, salt and black pepper in a bowl.
- Mix together chilled cauliflower, peas, chives, almonds and red onions in another bowl.
- Pour the dressing over this mixture and serve.

Nutrition: Calories: 203;Carbs: 7.6g;Fats: 18g;Proteins: 4.2g;Sodium: 28mg;Sugar: 2.9g

43) SPINACH AND BACON SALAD

Cooking Time: 15 Minutes **Servings: 4**

Ingredients:
- 2 eggs, boiled, halved, and sliced
- 10 oz. organic baby spinach, rinsed, and dried
- 8 pieces thick bacon, cooked and sliced
- ½ cup plain mayonnaise
- ½ medium red onion, thinly sliced

Directions:
- Mix together the mayonnaise and spinach in a large bowl.
- Stir in the rest of the ingredients and combine well.
- Dish out in a glass bowl and serve well.

Nutrition: Calories: 373;Carbs: ;Fats: 34.5g;Proteins: 11g;Sodium: 707mg;Sugar: 1.1g

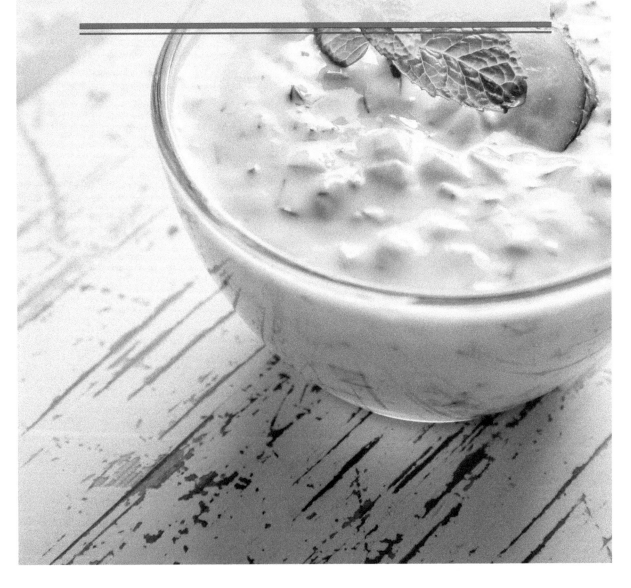

SAUCES & DRESSINGS

44) GREEK-STYLE CHICKEN AND POTATOES

Preparation Time: 10 minutes   **Cooking Time:** 50 minutes   **Servings: 4**

Ingredients:

- ✓ 4 lb chicken thighs 2 tbsp oregano
- ✓ 1 tbsp salt
- ✓ 1 tsp black pepper
- ✓ 2/3 cup chicken stock
- ✓ One pinch of cayenne pepper
- ✓ 1 tsp rosemary
- ✓ ½ cup lemon juice
- ✓ Six minced garlic cloves
- ✓ ½ cup olive oil
- ✓ Three sliced russet potatoes
- ✓ 1 tbsp chopped oregano

Directions:

- ❖ Add lemon juice, oregano, oil, cayenne pepper, salt, garlic, rosemary, black pepper potatoes, and chicken in a bowl. Mix them to coat everything well.
- ❖ Place chicken in a roasting tray.
- ❖ Spread potato pieces, 2/3 cup of stock, and marinade over chicken pieces.
- ❖ Bake in a preheated oven at 425 degrees for 20 minutes.
- ❖ Change the sides of the chicken and bake for 20 more minutes.
- ❖ Bake until chicken is done and shift chicken in serving dish.
- ❖ Mix potatoes with remaining juice and broil for three minutes.
- ❖ Shift the potatoes in the serving dish beside the chicken.
- ❖ Concentrate chicken stock left in a roasting tray on the stove over medium flame.

Nutrition: Calories: 138 kcal Fat: 74.5 g Protein: 80.4 g Carbs: 34.4 g Fiber: 3 g

45) ITALIAN BAKED FISH

Preparation Time: 5 minutes   **Cooking Time:** 30 minutes   **Servings: 6**

Ingredients:

- ✓ 1/3 cup olive oil
- ✓ Two diced tomatoes 1.5 chopped red onion
- ✓ Ten chopped garlic cloves
- ✓ 1 tsp Spanish paprika 2 tsp coriander
- ✓ 1 tsp cumin
- ✓ 1.5 tbsp capers
- ✓ ½ tsp cayenne pepper
- ✓ Salt to taste
- ✓ 1/3 cup raisins
- ✓ 1 tbsp of lemon juice
- ✓ Black pepper to taste
- ✓ Parsley for garnishing
- ✓ Zest of one lemon
- ✓ 1.5 lb white fish fillet
- ✓ Mint for garnishing

Directions:

- ❖ Cook onions in heated olive oil in a saucepan for three minutes.
- ❖ Stir in tomatoes, salt, capers, garlic, raisins, and spices and let them boil.
- ❖ Reduce the flame to low and simmer for 15 minutes.
- ❖ Rub fish with pepper and salt and set aside.
- ❖ Transfer half of the cooked tomato mixture to the baking pan, followed by fish, lemon juice, zest, and leftover tomato mixture.
- ❖ Bake in a preheated oven at 400 degrees for 18 minutes.
- ❖ Sprinkle mint and parsley and serve.

Nutrition: Calories: 308 kcal Fat: 17.4 g Protein: 27 g Carbs: 13.3 g Fiber: 2 g

46) GREEK TZATZIKI SAUCE AND DIP

Preparation Time: 10 minutes   **Cooking Time:** 0 minute   **Servings: 4**

Ingredients:

- ✓ ½ halved cucumber
- ✓ 3/4 cup Yogurt
- ✓ Two minced garlic cloves 2 tbsp red wine vinegar
- ✓ 1 tbsp minced dill
- ✓ One pinch of kosher salt
- ✓ One pinch of black pepper

Directions:

- ❖ Place dried shredded cucumber in a bowl.
- ❖ Mix garlic, vinegar, salt, yogurt, dill, and pepper in cucumber and mix well.
- ❖ Cover the bowl and place it in the refrigerator. The Tzatziki sauce is ready.
- ❖ Can store up to three days.

Nutrition: Calories: 30 kcal Fat: 1 g Protein: 4 g Carbs: 3 g Fiber: 1 g

47) ITALIAN PESTO AND GARLIC SHRIMP BRUSCHETTA

Preparation Time: 10 minutes   **Cooking Time:** 15 minutes   **Servings: 12**

Ingredients:

- ✓ 8 oz shrimp
- ✓ Black pepper to taste
- ✓ 2 tbsp butter
- ✓ 4 tbsp olive oil
- ✓ 20 basil leaves One bread
- ✓ Four minced garlic cloves 3 oz pesto
- ✓ 2 oz capers 3 oz sun-dried tomatoes
- ✓ 1 oz feta cheese
- ✓ kosher salt to taste
- ✓ Glaze Balsamic for garnishing

Directions:

- ❖ Sprinkle salt and pepper over shrimps in a bowl. Set aside for ten minutes.
- ❖ Add olive oil and butter of about 2 tbsp each in the pan and cook for 2 minutes over medium flame.
- ❖ Stir in garlic and sauté for one more minute.
- ❖ Mix shrimps and cook for four minutes.
- ❖ Remove from flame and let it set.
- ❖ Slice the bread and place in a baking tray and drizzle oil and toast in the oven for five minutes.
- ❖ Spread pesto sauce over each bread slice followed by sun-dried tomatoes, shrimp, caper, cheese, basil, and balsamic glaze and serve.

Nutrition: Calories: 168 kcal Fat: 7 g Protein: 5 g Carbs: 19 g Fiber: 1 g

48) EASY PAN-SEARED CITRUS SHRIMP

Preparation Time: 5 minutes **Cooking Time:** 10 minutes **Servings:** 6

Ingredients:
- ✓ 1 tbsp olive oil
- ✓ 6 tbsp cup lemon juice
- ✓ 1 cup of orange juice
- ✓ One sliced orange
- ✓ Five minced garlic cloves
- ✓ 1 tbsp chopped parsley
- ✓ 1 tbsp chopped red onion
- ✓ One pinch of red pepper flakes
- ✓ Kosher salt to taste
- ✓ Black pepper to taste 3 lb shrimp
- ✓ One wedge cut lemon

Directions:
- ❖ Mix parsley, pepper flakes, orange juice, oil, garlic, lemon juice, and onions in a bowl.
- ❖ Transfer the onion mixture to skillet and cook over medium flame for eight minutes.
- ❖ Add salt, pepper, and shrimps in a skillet and cook for five minutes or until shrimps are done.
- ❖ Garnish with parsley and lemon slices and serve.

Nutrition: Calories: 291 kcal Fat: 6 g Protein: 47 g Carbs: 11 g Fiber: 1 g

49) SIMPLE CUCUMBER AND TOMATO SALAD

Preparation Time: 10 minutes **Cooking Time:** 0 minute **Servings:** 4

Ingredients:
- ✓ One sliced English cucumber
- ✓ ½ sliced red onion
- ✓ Three diced tomatoes
- ✓ 2 tbsp olive oil
- ✓ Salt to taste
- ✓ 1 tbsp red wine vinegar
- ✓ Black pepper to taste

Directions:
- ❖ In a large mixing bowl, mix all the ingredients and place in the refrigerator for 20 minutes.
- ❖ Serve and enjoy it.

Nutrition: Calories: 104 kcal Fat: 8 g Protein: 2 g Carbs: 7 g Fiber: 2 g

50) EASY CITRUS AVOCADO DIP

Preparation Time: 15 minutes **Cooking Time:** 0 minute **Servings:** 8

Ingredients:
- ✓ Two diced oranges
- ✓ ½ cup chopped onions
- ✓ ½ cup chopped mint
- ✓ ½ cup chopped cilantro
- ✓ Olive oil as required
- ✓ Two sliced avocados
- ✓ ½ cup chopped walnuts
- ✓ Black pepper to taste
- ✓ Cayenne as required
- ✓ Salt to taste
- ✓ 1 tbsp of lime juice
- ✓ ¾ tsp sumac
- ✓ 1.75 oz shredded feta cheese

Directions:
- ❖ In a bowl, combine all the ingredients and mix well.
- ❖ Serve and enjoy it.

Nutrition: Calories: 147 kcal Fat: 10.3 g Protein: 2.8 g Carbs: 14.6 g Fiber: 2.1 g

51) TOMATOES ROAST WITH THYME AND FETA

Preparation Time: 5 minutes **Cooking Time:** 20 minutes **Servings:** 4

Ingredients:
- ✓ ½ tsp dried thyme
- ✓ 16 oz cherry tomatoes
- ✓ Black pepper to taste
- ✓ 3 tbsp olive oil
- ✓ Salt to taste
- ✓ 6 tbsp feta cheese

Directions:
- ❖ In a baking tray, put tomatoes.
- ❖ Pour olive oil and drizzle pepper, thyme leaves, and salt over tomatoes and mix well.
- ❖ Bake in a preheated oven at 450 degrees for 15 minutes.
- ❖ Drizzle cheese and broil for five minutes and serve when the cheese melts.

Nutrition: Calories: 195 kcal Fat: 7.3 g Protein: 2 g Carbs: 3.1 g Fiber: 1.1 g

52) GREEK-STYLE CHICKEN AND POTATOES

Preparation Time: 10 minutes   **Cooking Time:** 50 minutes   **Servings:** 4

Ingredients:

- ✓ 4 lb chicken thighs 2 tbsp oregano
- ✓ 1 tbsp salt
- ✓ 1 tsp black pepper
- ✓ 2/3 cup chicken stock
- ✓ One pinch of cayenne pepper
- ✓ 1 tsp rosemary
- ✓ ½ cup lemon juice
- ✓ Six minced garlic cloves
- ✓ ½ cup olive oil
- ✓ Three sliced russet potatoes
- ✓ 1 tbsp chopped oregano

Directions:

- ❖ Add lemon juice, oregano, oil, cayenne pepper, salt, garlic, rosemary, black pepper potatoes, and chicken in a bowl. Mix them to coat everything well.
- ❖ Place chicken in a roasting tray.
- ❖ Spread potato pieces, 2/3 cup of stock, and marinade over chicken pieces.
- ❖ Bake in a preheated oven at 425 degrees for 20 minutes.
- ❖ Change the sides of the chicken and bake for 20 more minutes.
- ❖ Bake until chicken is done and shift chicken in serving dish.
- ❖ Mix potatoes with remaining juice and broil for three minutes.
- ❖ Shift the potatoes in the serving dish beside the chicken.
- ❖ Concentrate chicken stock left in a roasting tray on the stove over medium flame.

Nutrition: Calories: 138 kcal Fat: 74.5 g Protein: 80.4 g Carbs: 34.4 g Fiber: 3 g

53) ITALIAN BAKED FISH

Preparation Time: 5 minutes   **Cooking Time:** 30 minutes   **Servings:** 6

Ingredients:

- ✓ 1/3 cup olive oil
- ✓ Two diced tomatoes 1.5 chopped red onion
- ✓ Ten chopped garlic cloves
- ✓ 1 tsp Spanish paprika 2 tsp coriander
- ✓ 1 tsp cumin
- ✓ 1.5 tbsp capers
- ✓ ½ tsp cayenne pepper
- ✓ Salt to taste
- ✓ 1/3 cup raisins
- ✓ 1 tbsp of lemon juice
- ✓ Black pepper to taste
- ✓ Parsley for garnishing
- ✓ Zest of one lemon
- ✓ 1.5 lb white fish fillet
- ✓ Mint for garnishing

Directions:

- ❖ Cook onions in heated olive oil in a saucepan for three minutes.
- ❖ Stir in tomatoes, salt, capers, garlic, raisins, and spices and let them boil.
- ❖ Reduce the flame to low and simmer for 15 minutes.
- ❖ Rub fish with pepper and salt and set aside.
- ❖ Transfer half of the cooked tomato mixture to the baking pan, followed by fish, lemon juice, zest, and leftover tomato mixture.
- ❖ Bake in a preheated oven at 400 degrees for 18 minutes.
- ❖ Sprinkle mint and parsley and serve.

Nutrition: Calories: 308 kcal Fat: 17.4 g Protein: 27 g Carbs: 13.3 g Fiber: 2 g

54) GREEK TZATZIKI SAUCE AND DIP

Preparation Time: 10 minutes   **Cooking Time:** 0 minute   **Servings:** 4

Ingredients:

- ✓ ½ halved cucumber
- ✓ 3/4 cup Yogurt
- ✓ Two minced garlic cloves 2 tbsp red wine vinegar
- ✓ 1 tbsp minced dill
- ✓ One pinch of kosher salt
- ✓ One pinch of black pepper

Directions:

- ❖ Place dried shredded cucumber in a bowl.
- ❖ Mix garlic, vinegar, salt, yogurt, dill, and pepper in cucumber and mix well.
- ❖ Cover the bowl and place it in the refrigerator. The Tzatziki sauce is ready.
- ❖ Can store up to three days.

Nutrition: Calories: 30 kcal Fat: 1 g Protein: 4 g Carbs: 3 g Fiber: 1 g

55) ITALIAN PESTO AND GARLIC SHRIMP BRUSCHETTA

Preparation Time: 10 minutes   **Cooking Time:** 15 minutes   **Servings:** 12

Ingredients:

- ✓ 8 oz shrimp
- ✓ Black pepper to taste
- ✓ 2 tbsp butter
- ✓ 4 tbsp olive oil
- ✓ 20 basil leaves One bread
- ✓ Four minced garlic cloves 3 oz pesto
- ✓ 2 oz capers 3 oz sun-dried tomatoes
- ✓ 1 oz feta cheese
- ✓ kosher salt to taste
- ✓ Glaze Balsamic for garnishing

Directions:

- ❖ Sprinkle salt and pepper over shrimps in a bowl. Set aside for ten minutes.
- ❖ Add olive oil and butter of about 2 tbsp each in the pan and cook for 2 minutes over medium flame.
- ❖ Stir in garlic and sauté for one more minute.
- ❖ Mix shrimps and cook for four minutes.
- ❖ Remove from flame and let it set.
- ❖ Slice the bread and place in a baking tray and drizzle oil and toast in the oven for five minutes.
- ❖ Spread pesto sauce over each bread slice followed by sun-dried tomatoes, shrimp, caper, cheese, basil, and balsamic glaze and serve.

Nutrition: Calories: 168 kcal Fat: 7 g Protein: 5 g Carbs: 19 g Fiber: 1 g

56) EASY PAN-SEARED CITRUS SHRIMP

Preparation Time: 5 minutes   **Cooking Time:** 10 minutes   **Servings:** 6

Ingredients:

- ✓ 1 tbsp olive oil
- ✓ 6 tbsp cup lemon juice
- ✓ 1 cup of orange juice
- ✓ One sliced orange
- ✓ Five minced garlic cloves
- ✓ 1 tbsp chopped parsley
- ✓ 1 tbsp chopped red onion
- ✓ One pinch of red pepper flakes
- ✓ Kosher salt to taste
- ✓ Black pepper to taste 3 lb shrimp
- ✓ One wedge cut lemon

Directions:

- ❖ Mix parsley, pepper flakes, orange juice, oil, garlic, lemon juice, and onions in a bowl.
- ❖ Transfer the onion mixture to skillet and cook over medium flame for eight minutes.
- ❖ Add salt, pepper, and shrimps in a skillet and cook for five minutes or until shrimps are done.
- ❖ Garnish with parsley and lemon slices and serve.

Nutrition: Calories: 291 kcal Fat: 6 g Protein: 47 g Carbs: 11 g Fiber: 1 g

57) SIMPLE CUCUMBER AND TOMATO SALAD

Preparation Time: 10 minutes   **Cooking Time:** 0 minute   **Servings:** 4

Ingredients:

- ✓ One sliced English cucumber
- ✓ ½ sliced red onion
- ✓ Three diced tomatoes
- ✓ 2 tbsp olive oil
- ✓ Salt to taste
- ✓ 1 tbsp red wine vinegar
- ✓ Black pepper to taste

Directions:

- ❖ In a large mixing bowl, mix all the ingredients and place in the refrigerator for 20 minutes.
- ❖ Serve and enjoy it.

Nutrition: Calories: 104 kcal Fat: 8 g Protein: 2 g Carbs: 7 g Fiber: 2 g

58) EASY CITRUS AVOCADO DIP

Preparation Time: 15 minutes   **Cooking Time:** 0 minute   **Servings:** 8

Ingredients:

- ✓ Two diced oranges
- ✓ ½ cup chopped onions
- ✓ ½ cup chopped mint
- ✓ ½ cup chopped cilantro
- ✓ Olive oil as required
- ✓ Two sliced avocados
- ✓ ½ cup chopped walnuts
- ✓ Black pepper to taste
- ✓ Cayenne as required
- ✓ Salt to taste
- ✓ 1 tbsp of lime juice
- ✓ ¾ tsp sumac
- ✓ 1.75 oz shredded feta cheese

Directions:

- ❖ In a bowl, combine all the ingredients and mix well.
- ❖ Serve and enjoy it.

Nutrition: Calories: 147 kcal Fat: 10.3 g Protein: 2.8 g Carbs: 14.6 g Fiber: 2.1 g

59) TOMATOES ROAST WITH THYME AND FETA

Preparation Time: 5 minutes   **Cooking Time:** 20 minutes   **Servings:** 4

Ingredients:

- ✓ ½ tsp dried thyme
- ✓ 16 oz cherry tomatoes
- ✓ Black pepper to taste
- ✓ 3 tbsp olive oil
- ✓ Salt to taste
- ✓ 6 tbsp feta cheese

Directions:

- ❖ In a baking tray, put tomatoes.
- ❖ Pour olive oil and drizzle pepper, thyme leaves, and salt over tomatoes and mix well.
- ❖ Bake in a preheated oven at 450 degrees for 15 minutes.
- ❖ Drizzle cheese and broil for five minutes and serve when the cheese melts.

Nutrition: Calories: 195 kcal Fat: 7.3 g Protein: 2 g Carbs: 3.1 g Fiber: 1.1 g

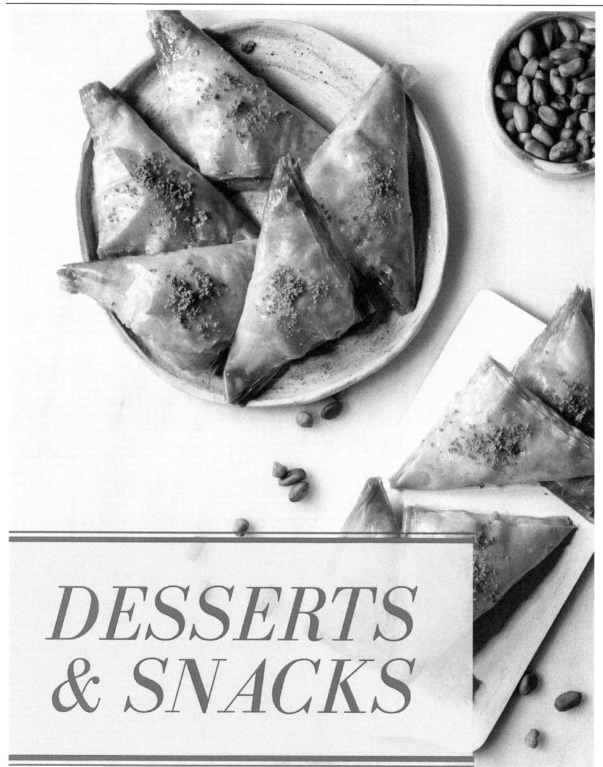

DESSERTS & SNACKS

60) SPECIAL CHUNKY MONKEY TRAIL MIX

Cooking Time: 1 Hour 30 Minutes   **Servings:** 6

Ingredients:

- ✓ 1 cup cashews, halved
- ✓ 2 cups raw walnuts, chopped or halved
- ✓ ⅓ cup coconut sugar
- ✓ ½ cup of chocolate chips
- ✓ 1 tsp vanilla extract
- ✓ 1 cup coconut flakes, unsweetened and make sure you have big flakes and not shredded
- ✓ 6 ounces dried banana slices
- ✓ 1 ½ tsp coconut oil at room temperature

Directions:

- ❖ Turn your crockpot to high and add the cashews, walnuts, vanilla, coconut oil, and sugar. Combine until the ingredients are well mixed and then cook for 45 minutes.
- ❖ Reduce the temperature on your crockpot to low.
- ❖ Continue to cook the mixture for another 20 minutes.
- ❖ Place a piece of parchment paper on your counter.
- ❖ Once the mix is done cooking, remove it from the crockpot and set on top of the parchment paper.
- ❖ Let the mixture sit and cool for 20 minutes.
- ❖ Pour the contents into a bowl and add the dried bananas and chocolate chips. Gently mix the ingredients together. You can store the mixture in Ziplock bags for a quick and easy snack.

Nutrition: calories: 250, fats: 6 grams, carbohydrates: 1grams, protein: 4 grams

61) DELICIOUS FIG-PECAN ENERGY BITES

Cooking Time: 20 Minutes   **Servings:** 6

Ingredients:

- ✓ ½ cup chopped pecans
- ✓ 2 tbsp honey
- ✓ ¾ cup dried figs, about 6 to 8, diced
- ✓ 2 tbsp wheat flaxseed
- ✓ ¼ cup quick oats
- ✓ 2 tbsp regular or powdered peanut butter

Directions:

- ❖ Combine the figs, quick oats, pecans, peanut butter, and flaxseed into a bowl. Stir the ingredients well.
- ❖ Drizzle honey onto the ingredients and mix everything with a wooden spoon. Do your best to press all the ingredients into the honey as you are stirring. If you start to struggle because the mixture is too sticky, set it in the freezer for 3 to 5 minutes.
- ❖ Divide the mixture into four sections.
- ❖ Take a wet rag and get your hands damp. You don't want them too wet or they won't work well with the mixture.
- ❖ Divide each of the four sections into 3 separate sections.
- ❖ Take one of the three sections and roll them up. Repeat with each section so you have a dozen energy bites once you are done.
- ❖ If you want to firm them up, you can place them into the freezer for a few minutes. Otherwise, you can enjoy them as soon as they are little energy balls.
- ❖ To store them, you'll want to keep them in a sealed container and set them in the fridge. They can be stored for about a week.

Nutrition: calories: 157, fats: 6 grams, carbohydrates: 26 grams, protein: 3 grams

62) MEDITERRANEAN STYLE BAKED APPLES

Cooking Time: 25 Minutes   **Servings:** 4

Ingredients:

- ✓ ½ lemon, squeezed for juice
- ✓ 1 ½ pounds of peeled and sliced apples
- ✓ ¼ tsp cinnamon

Directions:

- ❖ Set the temperature of your oven to 350 degrees Fahrenheit so it can preheat.
- ❖ Take a piece of parchment paper and lay on top of a baking pan.
- ❖ Combine your lemon juice, cinnamon, and apples into a medium bowl and mix well.
- ❖ Pour the apples onto the baking pan and arrange them so they are not doubled up.
- ❖ Place the pan in the oven and set your timer to 2minutes. The apples should be tender but not mushy.
- ❖ Remove from the oven, plate and enjoy!

Nutrition: calories: 90, fats: 0.3 grams, carbohydrates: 24 grams, protein: 0.5 grams

63) LOVELY STRAWBERRY POPSICLE

Cooking Time: 10 Minutes   **Servings: 5**

Ingredients:

- ✓ ½ cup almond milk
- ✓ 1 ½ cups fresh strawberries

Directions:

- ❖ Using a blender or hand mixer, combine the almond milk and strawberries thoroughly in a bowl.
- ❖ Using popsicle molds, pour the mixture into the molds and place the sticks into the mixture.
- ❖ Set in the freezer for at least 4 hours.
- ❖ Serve and enjoy—especially on a hot day!

Nutrition: calories: 3 fats: 0.5 grams, carbohydrates: 7 grams, protein: 0.6 grams.

64) SPECIAL FROZEN BLUEBERRY YOGURT

Cooking Time: 30 Minutes   **Servings: 6**

Ingredients:

- ✓ ⅔ cup honey
- ✓ 2 cups chilled yogurt
- ✓ 1 pint fresh blueberries
- ✓ 1 juiced and zested lime or lemon. You can even substitute an orange if your tastes prefer.

Directions:

- ❖ With a saucepan on your burner set to medium heat, add the honey, juiced fruit, zest, and blueberries.
- ❖ Stir the mixture continuously as it begins to simmer for 15 minutes.
- ❖ When the liquid is nearly gone, pour the contents into a bowl and place in the fridge for several minutes. You will want to stir the ingredients and check to see if they are chilled.
- ❖ Once the fruit is chilled, combine with the yogurt.
- ❖ Mix until the ingredients are well incorporated and enjoy.

Nutrition: calories: 233, fats: 3 grams, carbohydrates: 52 grams, protein: 3.5 grams

65) Cherry Brownies and Walnuts

Cooking Time: 25 To 30 Minutes   **Servings: 9**

Ingredients:

- ✓ 9 fresh cherries that are stemmed and pitted or 9 frozen cherries
- ✓ ½ cup sugar or sweetener substitute
- ✓ ¼ cup extra virgin olive oil
- ✓ 1 tsp vanilla extract
- ✓ ¼ tsp sea salt
- ✓ ½ cup whole-wheat pastry flour
- ✓ ¼ tsp baking powder
- ✓ ⅓ cup walnuts, chopped
- ✓ 2 eggs
- ✓ ½ cup plain Greek yogurt
- ✓ ⅓ cup cocoa powder, unsweetened

Directions:

- ❖ Make sure one of the metal racks in your oven is set in the middle.
- ❖ Turn the temperature on your oven to 375 degrees Fahrenheit.
- ❖ Using cooking spray, grease a 9-inch square pan.
- ❖ Take a large bowl and add the oil and sugar or sweetener substitute. Whisk the ingredients well.
- ❖ Add the eggs and use a mixer to beat the ingredients together.
- ❖ Pour in the yogurt and continue to beat the mixture until it is smooth.
- ❖ Take a medium bowl and combine the cocoa powder, flour, sea salt, and baking powder by whisking them together.
- ❖ Combine the powdered ingredients into the wet ingredients and use your electronic mixer to incorporate the ingredients together thoroughly.
- ❖ Add in the walnuts and stir.
- ❖ Pour the mixture into the pan.
- ❖ Sprinkle the cherries on top and push them into the batter. You can use any design, but it is best to make three rows and three columns with the cherries. This ensures that each piece of the brownie will have one cherry.
- ❖ Put the batter into the oven and turn your timer to 20 minutes.
- ❖ Check that the brownies are done using the toothpick test before removing them from the oven. Push the toothpick into the middle of the brownies and once it comes out clean, remove the brownies.
- ❖ Let the brownies cool for 5 to 10 minutes before cutting and serving.

Nutrition: calories: 225, fats: 10 grams, carbohydrates: 30 grams, protein: 5 grams

66) SPECIAL FRUIT DIP

Cooking Time: 10 To 15 Minutes   **Servings: 10**

Ingredients:

- ✓ ¼ cup coconut milk, full-fat is best
- ✓ ¼ cup vanilla yogurt
- ✓ ⅓ cup marshmallow creme
- ✓ 1 cup cream cheese, set at room temperature
- ✓ 2 tbsp maraschino cherry juice

Directions:

- ❖ In a large bowl, add the coconut milk, vanilla yogurt, marshmallow creme, cream cheese, and cherry juice.
- ❖ Using an electric mixer, set to low speed and blend the ingredients together until the fruit dip is smooth.
- ❖ Serve the dip with some of your favorite fruits and enjoy!

Nutrition: calories: 110, fats: 11 grams, carbohydrates: 3 grams, protein: 3 grams

67) Delicious Almond Shortbread Cookies

Cooking Time: 25 Minutes   **Servings: 16**

Ingredients:

- ✓ ½ cup coconut oil
- ✓ 1 tsp vanilla extract
- ✓ 2 egg yolks
- ✓ 1 tbsp brandy
- ✓ 1 cup powdered sugar
- ✓ 1 cup finely ground almonds
- ✓ 3 ½ cups cake flour
- ✓ ½ cup almond butter
- ✓ 1 tbsp water or rose flower water

Directions:

- ❖ In a large bowl, combine the coconut oil, powdered sugar, and butter. If the butter is not soft, you want to wait until it softens up. Use an electric mixer to beat the ingredients together at high speed.
- ❖ In a small bowl, add the egg yolks, brandy, water, and vanilla extract. Whisk well.
- ❖ Fold the egg yolk mixture into the large bowl.
- ❖ Add the flour and almonds. Fold and mix with a wooden spoon.
- ❖ Place the mixture into the fridge for at least 1 hour and 30 minutes.
- ❖ Preheat your oven to 325 degrees Fahrenheit.
- ❖ Take the mixture, which now looks like dough, and divide it into 1-inch balls.
- ❖ With a piece of parchment paper on a baking sheet, arrange the cookies and flatten them with a fork or your fingers.
- ❖ Place the cookies in the oven for 13 minutes, but watch them so they don't burn.
- ❖ Transfer the cookies onto a rack to cool for a couple of minutes before enjoying!

Nutrition: calories: 250, fats: 14 grams, carbohydrates: 30 grams, protein: 3 grams

68) CLASSIC CHOCOLATE FRUIT KEBABS

Cooking Time: 30 Minutes   **Servings: 6**

Ingredients:

- ✓ 24 blueberries
- ✓ 12 strawberries with the green leafy top part removed
- ✓ 12 green or red grapes, seedless
- ✓ 12 pitted cherries
- ✓ 8 ounces chocolate

Directions:

- ❖ Line a baking sheet with a piece of parchment paper and place 6, -inch long wooden skewers on top of the paper.
- ❖ Start by threading a piece of fruit onto the skewers. You can create and follow any pattern that you like with the ingredients. An example pattern is 1 strawberry, 1 cherry, blueberries, 2 grapes. Repeat the pattern until all of the fruit is on the skewers.
- ❖ In a saucepan on medium heat, melt the chocolate. Stir continuously until the chocolate has melted completely.
- ❖ Carefully scoop the chocolate into a plastic sandwich bag and twist the bag closed starting right above the chocolate.
- ❖ Snip the corner of the bag with scissors.
- ❖ Drizzle the chocolate onto the kebabs by squeezing it out of the bag.
- ❖ Put the baking pan into the freezer for 20 minutes.
- ❖ Serve and enjoy!

Nutrition: calories: 254, fats: 15 grams, carbohydrates: 28 grams, protein: 4 grams *69)*

70) MEDITERRANEAN-STYLE BLACKBERRY ICE CREAM

Cooking Time: 15 Minutes   **Servings:** 6

Ingredients:
- ✓ 3 egg yolks
- ✓ 1 container of Greek yogurt
- ✓ 1 pound mashed blackberries
- ✓ ½ tsp vanilla essence
- ✓ 1 tsp arrowroot powder
- ✓ ¼ tsp ground cloves
- ✓ 5 ounces sugar or sweetener substitute
- ✓ 1 pound heavy cream

Directions:
- ❖ In a small bowl, add the arrowroot powder and egg yolks. Whisk or beat them with an electronic mixture until they are well combined.
- ❖ Set a saucepan on top of your stove and turn your heat to medium.
- ❖ Add the heavy cream and bring it to a boil.
- ❖ Turn off the heat and add the egg mixture into the cream through folding.
- ❖ Turn the heat back on to medium and pour in the sugar. Cook the mixture for 10 minutes or until it starts to thicken.
- ❖ Remove the mixture from heat and place it in the fridge so it can completely cool. This should take about one hour.
- ❖ Once the mixture is cooled, add in the Greek yogurt, ground cloves, blackberries, and vanilla by folding in the ingredients.
- ❖ Transfer the ice cream into a container and place it in the freezer for at least two hours.
- ❖ Serve and enjoy!

Nutrition: calories: 402, fats: 20 grams, carbohydrates: 52 grams, protein: 8 grams

71) CLASSIC STUFFED FIGS

Cooking Time: 20 Minutes   **Servings:** 6

Ingredients:
- ✓ 10 halved fresh figs
- ✓ 20 chopped almonds
- ✓ 4 ounces goat cheese, divided
- ✓ 2 tbsp of raw honey

Directions:
- ❖ Turn your oven to broiler mode and set it to a high temperature.
- ❖ Place your figs, cut side up, on a baking sheet. If you like to place a piece of parchment paper on top you can do this, but it is not necessary.
- ❖ Sprinkle each fig with half of the goat cheese.
- ❖ Add a tbsp of chopped almonds to each fig.
- ❖ Broil the figs for 3 to 4 minutes.
- ❖ Take them out of the oven and let them cool for 5 to 7 minutes.
- ❖ Sprinkle with the remaining goat cheese and honey.

72) PEACHES AND BLUE CHEESE CREAM

Cooking Time: 20 Hours 10 Minutes   **Servings:** 4

- ✓ ¼ tsp cardamom pods
- ✓ ⅔ cup red wine
- ✓ 2 tbsp honey, raw or your preferred variety
- ✓ 1 vanilla bean
- ✓ 1 tsp allspice berries
- ✓ 4 tbsp dried cherries

Directions:
- ❖ Set a saucepan on top of your stove range and add the cinnamon stick, cloves, orange juice, cardamom, vanilla, allspice, red wine, and orange zest. Whisk the ingredients well. Add your peaches to the mixture and poach them for hours or until they become soft.
- ❖ Take a spoon to remove the peaches and boil the rest of the liquid to make the syrup. You want the liquid to reduce itself by at least half.
- ❖ While the liquid is boiling, combine the dried cherries, blue cheese, and honey into a bowl. Once your peaches are cooled, slice them into halves.
- ❖ Top each peach with the blue cheese mixture and then drizzle the liquid onto the top. Serve and enjoy!

Nutrition: calories: 211, fats: 24 grams, carbohydrates: 15 grams, protein: 6 grams

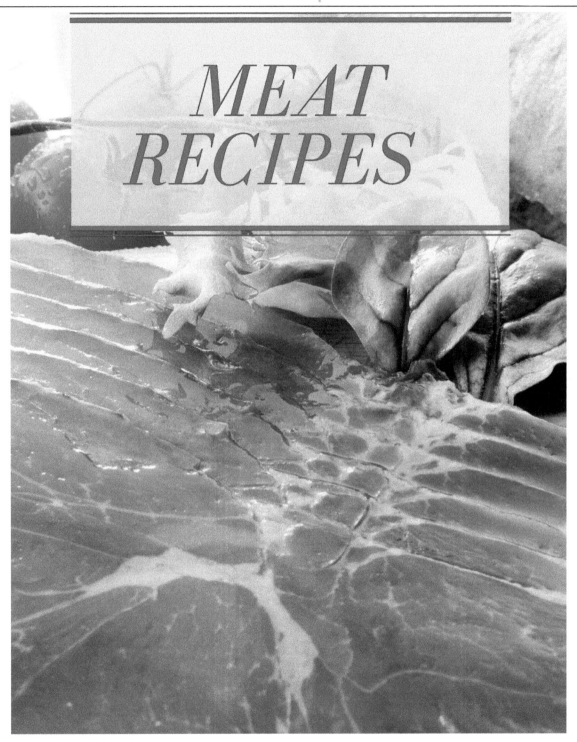

MEAT
RECIPES

73) SPECIAL GROUND PORK SKILLET

Cooking Time: 25 Minutes   **Servings:** 4

Ingredients:

- 1 ½ pounds ground pork
- 2 tbsp olive oil
- 1 bunch kale, trimmed and roughly chopped
- 1 cup onions, sliced
- 1/4 tsp black pepper, or more to taste
- 1/4 cup tomato puree
- 1 bell pepper, chopped
- 1 tsp sea salt
- 1 cup chicken bone broth
- 1/4 cup port wine
- 2 cloves garlic, pressed
- 1 chili pepper, sliced

Directions:

- ❖ Heat tbsp of the olive oil in a cast-iron skillet over a moderately high heat. Now, sauté the onion, garlic, and peppers until they are tender and fragrant; reserve.
- ❖ Heat the remaining tbsp of olive oil; once hot, cook the ground pork and approximately 5 minutes until no longer pink.
- ❖ Add in the other ingredients and continue to cook for 15 to 17 minutes or until cooked through.
- ❖ Storing
- ❖ Place the ground pork mixture in airtight containers or Ziploc bags; keep in your refrigerator for up to 3 to 4 days.
- ❖ For freezing, place the ground pork mixture in airtight containers or heavy-duty freezer bags. Freeze up to 2 to 3 months. Defrost in the refrigerator. Bon appétit!

Nutrition: 349 Calories; 13g Fat; 4.4g Carbs; 45.3g Protein; 1.2g Fiber

74) LOVELY CHEESY GREEK-STYLE PORK

Cooking Time: 20 Minutes   **Servings:** 6

Ingredients:

- 1 tbsp sesame oil
- 1 ½ pounds pork shoulder, cut into strips
- Himalayan salt and freshly ground black pepper, to taste
- 1/2 tsp cayenne pepper
- 1/2 cup shallots, roughly chopped
- 2 bell peppers, sliced
- 1/4 cup cream of onion soup
- 1/2 tsp Sriracha sauce
- 1 tbsp tahini (sesame butter
- 1 tbsp soy sauce
- 4 ounces gouda cheese, cut into small pieces

Directions:

- ❖ Heat he sesame oil in a wok over a moderately high flame.
- ❖ Stir-fry the pork strips for 3 to 4 minutes or until just browned on all sides. Add in the spices, shallots and bell peppers and continue to cook for a further 4 minutes.
- ❖ Stir in the cream of onion soup, Sriracha, sesame butter, and soy sauce; continue to cook for to 4 minutes more.
- ❖ Top with the cheese and continue to cook until the cheese has melted.
- ❖ Storing
- ❖ Place your stir-fry in six airtight containers or Ziploc bags; keep in your refrigerator for 3 to 4 days.
- ❖ For freezing, wrap tightly with heavy-duty aluminum foil or freezer wrap. It will maintain the best quality for 2 to 3 months. Defrost in the refrigerator and reheat in your wok.

Nutrition: 424 Calories; 29.4g Fat; 3. Carbs; 34.2g Protein; 0.6g Fiber

75) SPECIAL PORK IN BLUE CHEESE SAUCE

Cooking Time: 30 Minutes   **Servings:** 6

Ingredients:

- 2 pounds pork center cut loin roast, boneless and cut into 6 pieces
- 1 tbsp coconut aminos
- 6 ounces blue cheese
- 1/3 cup heavy cream
- 1/3 cup port wine
- 1/3 cup roasted vegetable broth, preferably homemade
- 1 tsp dried hot chile flakes
- 1 tsp dried rosemary
- 1 tbsp lard
- 1 shallot, chopped
- 2 garlic cloves, chopped
- Salt and freshly cracked black peppercorns, to taste

Directions:

- ❖ Rub each piece of the pork with salt, black peppercorns, and rosemary.
- ❖ Melt the lard in a saucepan over a moderately high flame. Sear the pork on all sides about 15 minutes; set aside.
- ❖ Cook the shallot and garlic until they've softened. Add in port wine to scrape up any brown bits from the bottom.
- ❖ Reduce the heat to medium-low and add in the remaining ingredients; continue to simmer until the sauce has thickened and reduced.
- ❖ Storing
- ❖ Divide the pork and sauce into six portions; place each portion in a separate airtight container or Ziploc bag; keep in your refrigerator for 3 to 4 days.
- ❖ Freeze the pork and sauce in airtight containers or heavy-duty freezer bags. Freeze up to 4 months. Defrost in the refrigerator. Bon appétit!

Nutrition: 34Calories; 18.9g Fat; 1.9g Carbs; 40.3g Protein; 0.3g Fiber

76) MISSISSIPPI-STYLE PULLED PORK

Cooking Time: 6 Hours   **Servings: 4**

Ingredients:

- ✓ 1 ½ pounds pork shoulder
- ✓ 1 tbsp liquid smoke sauce
- ✓ 1 tsp chipotle powder
- ✓ Au Jus gravy seasoning packet
- ✓ 2 onions, cut into wedges
- ✓ Kosher salt and freshly ground black pepper, taste

Directions:

- ❖ Mix the liquid smoke sauce, chipotle powder, Au Jus gravy seasoning packet, salt and pepper. Rub the spice mixture into the pork on all sides.
- ❖ Wrap in plastic wrap and let it marinate in your refrigerator for 3 hours.
- ❖ Prepare your grill for indirect heat. Place the pork butt roast on the grate over a drip pan and top with onions; cover the grill and cook for about 6 hours.
- ❖ Transfer the pork to a cutting board. Now, shred the meat into bite-sized pieces using two forks.
- ❖ Storing
- ❖ Divide the pork between four airtight containers or Ziploc bags; keep in your refrigerator for up to 3 to 5 days.
- ❖ For freezing, place the pork in airtight containers or heavy-duty freezer bags. Freeze up to 4 months. Defrost in the refrigerator. Bon appétit!

Nutrition: 350 Calories; 11g Fat; 5g Carbs; 53.6g Protein; 2.2g Fiber

77) SPICY WITH CHEESY TURKEY DIP

Cooking Time: 25 Minutes   **Servings: 4**

Ingredients:

- ✓ 1 Fresno chili pepper, deveined and minced
- ✓ 1 ½ cups Ricotta cheese, creamed, 4% fat, softened
- ✓ 1/4 cup sour cream
- ✓ 1 tbsp butter, room temperature
- ✓ 1 shallot, chopped
- ✓ 1 tsp garlic, pressed
- ✓ 1 pound ground turkey
- ✓ 1/2 cup goat cheese, shredded
- ✓ Salt and black pepper, to taste
- ✓ 1 ½ cups Gruyère, shredded

Directions:

- ❖ Melt the butter in a frying pan over a moderately high flame. Now, sauté the onion and garlic until they have softened.
- ❖ Stir in the ground turkey and continue to cook until it is no longer pink.
- ❖ Transfer the sautéed mixture to a lightly greased baking dish. Add in Ricotta, sour cream, goat cheese, salt, pepper, and chili pepper.
- ❖ Top with the shredded Gruyère cheese. Bake in the preheated oven at 350 degrees F for about 20 minutes or until hot and bubbly in top.
- ❖ Storing
- ❖ Place your dip in an airtight container; keep in your refrigerator for up 3 to 4 days. Enjoy!

Nutrition: 284 Calories; 19g Fat; 3.2g Carbs; 26. Protein; 1.6g Fiber

78) TURKEY CHORIZO AND BOK CHOY

Cooking Time: 50 Minutes   **Servings: 4**

Ingredients:

- ✓ 4 mild turkey Chorizo, sliced
- ✓ 1/2 cup full-fat milk
- ✓ 6 ounces Gruyère cheese, preferably freshly grated
- ✓ 1 yellow onion, chopped
- ✓ Coarse salt and ground black pepper, to taste
- ✓ 1 pound Bok choy, tough stem ends trimmed
- ✓ 1 cup cream of mushroom soup
- ✓ 1 tbsp lard, room temperature

Directions:

- ❖ Melt the lard in a nonstick skillet over a moderate flame; cook the Chorizo sausage for about 5 minutes, stirring occasionally to ensure even cooking; reserve.
- ❖ Add in the onion, salt, pepper, Bok choy, and cream of mushroom soup. Continue to cook for 4 minutes longer or until the vegetables have softened.
- ❖ Spoon the mixture into a lightly oiled casserole dish. Top with the reserved Chorizo.
- ❖ In a mixing bowl, thoroughly combine the milk and cheese. Pour the cheese mixture over the sausage.
- ❖ Cover with foil and bake at 36degrees F for about 35 minutes.
- ❖ Storing
- ❖ Cut your casserole into four portions. Place each portion in an airtight container; keep in your refrigerator for 3 to 4 days.
- ❖ For freezing, wrap your portions tightly with heavy-duty aluminum foil or freezer wrap. Freeze up to 1 to 2 months. Defrost in the refrigerator. Enjoy!

Nutrition: 18Calories; 12g Fat; 2.6g Carbs; 9.4g Protein; 1g Fiber

79) CLASSIC SPICY CHICKEN BREASTS

Cooking Time: 30 Minutes   **Servings: 6**

Ingredients:
- ✓ 1 ½ pounds chicken breasts
- ✓ 1 bell pepper, deveined and chopped
- ✓ 1 leek, chopped
- ✓ 1 tomato, pureed
- ✓ 2 tbsp coriander
- ✓ 2 garlic cloves, minced
- ✓ 1 tsp cayenne pepper
- ✓ 1 tsp dry thyme
- ✓ 1/4 cup coconut aminos
- ✓ Sea salt and ground black pepper, to taste

Directions:
- ❖ Rub each chicken breasts with the garlic, cayenne pepper, thyme, salt and black pepper. Cook the chicken in a saucepan over medium-high heat.
- ❖ Sear for about 5 minutes until golden brown on all sides.
- ❖ Fold in the tomato puree and coconut aminos and bring it to a boil. Add in the pepper, leek, and coriander.
- ❖ Reduce the heat to simmer. Continue to cook, partially covered, for about 20 minutes.
- ❖ Storing
- ❖ Place the chicken breasts in airtight containers or Ziploc bags; keep in your refrigerator for 3 to 4 days.
- ❖ For freezing, place the chicken breasts in airtight containers or heavy-duty freezer bags. It will maintain the best quality for about 4 months. Defrost in the refrigerator. Bon appétit!

Nutrition: 239 Calories; 6g Fat; 5.5g Carbs; 34.3g Protein; 1g Fiber

80) DELICIOUS SAUCY BOSTON BUTT

Cooking Time: 1 Hour 20 Minutes   **Servings: 8**

Ingredients:
- ✓ 1 tbsp lard, room temperature
- ✓ 2 pounds Boston butt, cubed
- ✓ Salt and freshly ground pepper
- ✓ 1/2 tsp mustard powder
- ✓ A bunch of spring onions, chopped
- ✓ 2 garlic cloves, minced
- ✓ 1/2 tbsp ground cardamom
- ✓ 2 tomatoes, pureed
- ✓ 1 bell pepper, deveined and chopped
- ✓ 1 jalapeno pepper, deveined and finely chopped
- ✓ 1/2 cup unsweetened coconut milk
- ✓ 2 cups chicken bone broth

Directions:
- ❖ In a wok, melt the lard over moderate heat. Season the pork belly with salt, pepper and mustard powder.
- ❖ Sear the pork for 8 to 10 minutes, stirring periodically to ensure even cooking; set aside, keeping it warm.
- ❖ In the same wok, sauté the spring onions, garlic, and cardamom. Spoon the sautéed vegetables along with the reserved pork into the slow cooker.
- ❖ Add in the remaining ingredients, cover with the lid and cook for 1 hour 10 minutes over low heat.
- ❖ Storing
- ❖ Divide the pork and vegetables between airtight containers or Ziploc bags; keep in your refrigerator for up to 3 to 5 days.
- ❖ For freezing, place the pork and vegetables in airtight containers or heavy-duty freezer bags. Freeze up to 4 months. Defrost in the refrigerator. Bon appétit!

Nutrition: 369 Calories; 20.2g Fat; 2.9g Carbs; 41.3g Protein; 0.7g Fiber

81) OLD-FASHIONED HUNGARIAN GOULASH

Cooking Time: 9 Hours 10 Minutes   **Servings: 4**

Ingredients:
- ✓ 1 ½ pounds pork butt, chopped
- ✓ 1 tsp sweet Hungarian paprika
- ✓ 2 Hungarian hot peppers, deveined and minced
- ✓ 1 cup leeks, chopped
- ✓ 1 ½ tbsp lard
- ✓ 1 tsp caraway seeds, ground
- ✓ 4 cups vegetable broth
- ✓ 2 garlic cloves, crushed
- ✓ 1 tsp cayenne pepper
- ✓ 2 cups tomato sauce with herbs
- ✓ 1 ½ pounds pork butt, chopped
- ✓ 1 tsp sweet Hungarian paprika
- ✓ 2 Hungarian hot peppers, deveined and minced
- ✓ 1 cup leeks, chopped
- ✓ 1 ½ tbsp lard
- ✓ 1 tsp caraway seeds, ground
- ✓ 4 cups vegetable broth
- ✓ 2 garlic cloves, crushed
- ✓ 1 tsp cayenne pepper
- ✓ 2 cups tomato sauce with herbs

Directions:
- ❖ Melt the lard in a heavy-bottomed pot over medium-high heat. Sear the pork for 5 to 6 minutes until just browned on all sides; set aside.
- ❖ Add in the leeks and garlic; continue to cook until they have softened.
- ❖ Place the reserved pork along with the sautéed mixture in your crock pot. Add in the other ingredients and stir to combine.
- ❖ Cover with the lid and slow cook for 9 hours on the lowest setting.
- ❖ Storing
- ❖ Spoon your goulash into four airtight containers or Ziploc bags; keep in your refrigerator for up to 3 to 4 days.
- ❖ For freezing, place the goulash in airtight containers. Freeze up to 4 to 6 months. Defrost in the refrigerator. Enjoy!

Nutrition: 456 Calories; 27g Fat; 6.7g Carbs; 32g Protein; 3.4g Fiber

82) FLATBREAD AND CHICKEN LIVER PÂTÉ

Cooking Time: 2 Hours 15 Minutes   **Servings:** 4

Ingredients:

- ✓ 1 yellow onion, finely chopped
- ✓ 10 ounces chicken livers
- ✓ 1/2 tsp Mediterranean seasoning blend
- ✓ 4 tbsp olive oil
- ✓ 1 garlic clove, minced

- ✓ For Flatbread:
- ✓ 1 cup lukewarm water
- ✓ 1/2 stick butter
- ✓ 1/2 cup flax meal
- ✓ 1 ½ tbsp psyllium husks
- ✓ 1 ¼ cups almond flour

Directions:

- ❖ Pulse the chicken livers along with the seasoning blend, olive oil, onion and garlic in your food processor; reserve.
- ❖ Mix the dry ingredients for the flatbread. Mix in all the wet ingredients. Whisk to combine well.
- ❖ Let it stand at room temperature for 2 hours. Divide the dough into 8 balls and roll them out on a flat surface.
- ❖ In a lightly greased pan, cook your flatbread for 1 minute on each side or until golden.
- ❖ Storing
- ❖ Wrap the chicken liver pate in foil before packing it into airtight containers; keep in your refrigerator for up to 7 days.
- ❖ For freezing, place the chicken liver pate in airtight containers or heavy-duty freezer bags. Freeze up to 2 months. Defrost overnight in the refrigerator.
- ❖ As for the keto flatbread, wrap them in foil before packing them into airtight containers; keep in your refrigerator for up to 4 days.
- ❖ Bon appétit!

Nutrition: 395 Calories; 30.2g Fat; 3.6g Carbs; 17.9g Protein; 0.5g Fiber

83) SATURDAY CHICKEN WITH CAULIFLOWER SALAD

Cooking Time: 20 Minutes   **Servings:** 2

Ingredients:

- ✓ 1 tsp hot paprika
- ✓ 2 tbsp fresh basil, snipped
- ✓ 1/2 cup mayonnaise
- ✓ 1 tsp mustard
- ✓ 2 tsp butter
- ✓ 2 chicken wings

- ✓ 1/2 cup cheddar cheese, shredded
- ✓ Sea salt and ground black pepper, to taste
- ✓ 2 tbsp dry sherry
- ✓ 1 shallot, finely minced
- ✓ 1/2 head of cauliflower

Directions:

- ❖ Boil the cauliflower in a pot of salted water until it has softened; cut into small florets and place in a salad bowl.
- ❖ Melt the butter in a saucepan over medium-high heat. Cook the chicken for about 8 minutes or until the skin is crisp and browned. Season with hot paprika salt, and black pepper.
- ❖ Whisk the mayonnaise, mustard, dry sherry, and shallot and dress your salad. Top with cheddar cheese and fresh basil.
- ❖ Storing
- ❖ Place the chicken wings in airtight containers or Ziploc bags; keep in your refrigerator for up 3 to 4 days.
- ❖ Keep the cauliflower salad in your refrigerator for up 3 days.
- ❖ For freezing, place the chicken wings in airtight containers or heavy-duty freezer bags. Freeze up to 3 months. Once thawed in the refrigerator, reheat in a saucepan until thoroughly warmed.

Nutrition: 444 Calories; 36g Fat; 5.7g Carbs; 20.6g Protein; 4.3g Fiber

84) SPECIAL KANSAS-STYLE MEATLOAF

Cooking Time: 1 Hour 10 Minutes   **Servings:** 8

Ingredients:

- ✓ 2 pounds ground pork
- ✓ 2 eggs, beaten
- ✓ 1/2 cup onions, chopped
- ✓ 1/2 cup marinara sauce, bottled
- ✓ 8 ounces Colby cheese, shredded
- ✓ 1 tsp granulated garlic

- ✓ Sea salt and freshly ground black pepper, to taste
- ✓ 1 tsp lime zest
- ✓ 1 tsp mustard seeds
- ✓ 1/2 cup tomato puree
- ✓ 1 tbsp Erythritol

Directions:

- ❖ Mix the ground pork with the eggs, onions, marinara salsa, cheese, granulated garlic, salt, pepper, lime zest, and mustard seeds; mix to combine.
- ❖ Press the mixture into a lightly-greased loaf pan. Mix the tomato paste with the Erythritol and spread the mixture over the top of your meatloaf.
- ❖ Bake in the preheated oven at 5 degrees F for about 1 hour 10 minutes, rotating the pan halfway through the cook time. Storing Wrap your meatloaf tightly with heavy-duty aluminum foil or plastic wrap. Then, keep in your refrigerator for up to 3 to 4 days.
- ❖ For freezing, wrap your meatloaf tightly to prevent freezer burn. Freeze up to 3 to 4 months. Defrost in the refrigerator. Bon appétit!

Nutrition: 318 Calories; 14. Fat; 6.2g Carbs; 39.3g Protein; 0.3g Fiber

85) ORIGINAL TURKEY KEBABS

Cooking Time: 30 Minutes   **Servings: 6**

Ingredients:
- ✓ 1 ½ pounds turkey breast, cubed
- ✓ 3 Spanish peppers, sliced
- ✓ 2 zucchinis, cut into thick slices
- ✓ 1 onion, cut into wedges
- ✓ 2 tbsp olive oil, room temperature
- ✓ 1 tbsp dry ranch seasoning

Directions:
- ❖ Thread the turkey pieces and vegetables onto bamboo skewers. Sprinkle the skewers with dry ranch seasoning and olive oil.
- ❖ Grill your kebabs for about 10 minutes, turning them periodically to ensure even cooking.
- ❖ Storing
- ❖ Wrap your kebabs in foil before packing them into airtight containers; keep in your refrigerator for up to 3 to 4 days.
- ❖ For freezing, place your kebabs in airtight containers or heavy-duty freezer bags. Freeze up to 2-3 months. Defrost in the refrigerator. Bon appétit!

Nutrition: 2 Calories; 13.8g Fat; 6.7g Carbs; 25.8g Protein; 1.2g Fiber

86) ORIGINAL MEXICAN-STYLE TURKEY BACON BITES

Cooking Time: 5 Minutes   **Servings: 4**

Ingredients:
- ✓ 4 ounces turkey bacon, chopped
- ✓ 4 ounces Neufchatel cheese
- ✓ 1 tbsp butter, cold
- ✓ 1 jalapeno pepper, deveined and minced
- ✓ 1 tsp Mexican oregano
- ✓ 2 tbsp scallions, finely chopped

Directions:
- ❖ Thoroughly combine all ingredients in a mixing bowl.
- ❖ Roll the mixture into 8 balls.
- ❖ Storing
- ❖ Divide the turkey bacon bites between two airtight containers or Ziploc bags; keep in your refrigerator for up 3 to days.

Nutrition: 19Calories; 16.7g Fat; 2.2g Carbs; 8.8g Protein; 0.3g Fiber

87) ORIGINAL MUFFINS WITH GROUND PORK

Cooking Time: 25 Minutes   **Servings: 6**

Ingredients:
- ✓ 1 stick butter
- ✓ 3 large eggs, lightly beaten
- ✓ 2 tbsp full-fat milk
- ✓ 1/2 tsp ground cardamom
- ✓ 3 ½ cups almond flour
- ✓ 2 tbsp flaxseed meal
- ✓ 1 tsp baking powder
- ✓ 2 cups ground pork
- ✓ Salt and pepper, to your liking
- ✓ 1/2 tsp dried basil

Directions:
- ❖ In the preheated frying pan, cook the ground pork until the juices run clear, approximately 5 minutes.
- ❖ Add in the remaining ingredients and stir until well combined.
- ❖ Spoon the mixture into lightly greased muffin cups. Bake in the preheated oven at 5 degrees F for about 17 minutes.
- ❖ Allow your muffins to cool down before unmolding and storing.
- ❖ Storing
- ❖ Place your muffins in the airtight containers or Ziploc bags; keep in the refrigerator for a week.
- ❖ For freezing, divide your muffins among Ziploc bags and freeze up to 3 months. Defrost in your microwave for a couple of minutes. Bon appétit!

Nutrition: 330 Calories; 30.3g Fat; 2.3g Carbs; 19g Protein; 1.2g Fiber

88) Authentic Pork Chops With Herbs

Cooking Time: 20 Minutes   **Servings: 4**

Ingredients:
- ✓ 1 tbsp butter
- ✓ 1 pound pork chops
- ✓ 2 rosemary sprigs, minced
- ✓ 1 tsp dried marjoram
- ✓ 1 tsp dried parsley
- ✓ A bunch of spring onions, roughly chopped
- ✓ 1 thyme sprig, minced
- ✓ 1/2 tsp granulated garlic
- ✓ 1/2 tsp paprika, crushed
- ✓ Coarse salt and ground black pepper, to taste

Directions:
- ❖ Season the pork chops with the granulated garlic, paprika, salt, and black pepper.
- ❖ Melt the butter in a frying pan over a moderate flame. Cook the pork chops for 6 to 8 minutes, turning them occasionally to ensure even cooking.
- ❖ Add in the remaining ingredients and cook an additional 4 minutes.
- ❖ Storing
- ❖ Divide the pork chops into four portions; place each portion in a separate airtight container or Ziploc bag; keep in your refrigerator for 3 to 4 days.
- ❖ Freeze the pork chops in airtight containers or heavy-duty freezer bags. Freeze up to 4 months. Defrost in the refrigerator. Bon appétit!

89) TYPICAL MEDITERRANEAN-STYLE CHEESY PORK LOIN

Cooking Time: 25 Minutes   **Servings: 4**

Ingredients:

- ✓ 1 pound pork loin, cut into 1-inch-thick pieces
- ✓ 1 tsp Mediterranean seasoning mix
- ✓ Salt and pepper, to taste
- ✓ 1 onion, sliced
- ✓ 1 tsp fresh garlic, smashed
- ✓ 2 tbsp black olives, pitted and sliced
- ✓ 2 tbsp balsamic vinegar
- ✓ 1/2 cup Romano cheese, grated
- ✓ 2 tbsp butter, room temperature
- ✓ 1 tbsp curry paste
- ✓ 1 cup roasted vegetable broth
- ✓ 1 tbsp oyster sauce

Directions:

- ❖ In a frying pan, melt the butter over a moderately high heat. Once hot, cook the pork until browned on all sides; season with salt and black pepper and set aside.
- ❖ In the pan drippings, cook the onion and garlic for 4 to 5 minutes or until they've softened.
- ❖ Add in the Mediterranean seasoning mix, curry paste, and vegetable broth. Continue to cook until the sauce has thickened and reduced slightly or about 10 minutes. Add in the remaining ingredients along with the reserved pork.
- ❖ Top with cheese and cook for 10 minutes longer or until cooked through.
- ❖ Storing
- ❖ Divide the pork loin between four airtight containers; keep in your refrigerator for 3 to 5 days.
- ❖ For freezing, place the pork loin in airtight containers or heavy-duty freezer bags. Freeze up to 4 to 6 months. Defrost in the refrigerator. Enjoy!

Nutrition: 476 Calories; 35.3g Fat; 6.2g Carbs; 31.1g Protein; 1.4g Fiber

90) OVEN-ROASTED SPARE RIBS

Cooking Time: 3 Hour 40 Minutes   **Servings: 6**

Ingredients:

- ✓ 2 pounds spare ribs
- ✓ 1 garlic clove, minced
- ✓ 1 tsp dried marjoram
- ✓ 1 lime, halved
- ✓ Salt and ground black pepper, to taste

Directions:

- ❖ Toss all ingredients in a ceramic dish.
- ❖ Cover and let it refrigerate for 5 to 6 hours.
- ❖ Roast the foil-wrapped ribs in the preheated oven at 275 degrees F degrees for about hours 30 minutes.
- ❖ Storing
- ❖ Divide the ribs into six portions. Place each portion of ribs in an airtight container; keep in your refrigerator for 3 to 3 days.
- ❖ For freezing, place the ribs in airtight containers or heavy-duty freezer bags. Freeze up to 4 to months. Defrost in the refrigerator and reheat in the preheated oven. Bon appétit!

Nutrition: 385 Calories; 29g Fat; 1.8g Carbs; 28.3g Protein; 0.1g Fiber

91) HEALTHY PARMESAN CHICKEN SALAD

Cooking Time: 20 Minutes   **Servings: 6**

Ingredients:

- ✓ 2 romaine hearts, leaves separated
- ✓ Flaky sea salt and ground black pepper, to taste
- ✓ 1/4 tsp chili pepper flakes
- ✓ 1 tsp dried basil
- ✓ 1/4 cup Parmesan, finely grated
- ✓ 2 chicken breasts
- ✓ 2 Lebanese cucumbers, sliced
- ✓ For the dressing:
- ✓ 2 large egg yolks
- ✓ 1 tsp Dijon mustard
- ✓ 1 tbsp fresh lemon juice
- ✓ 1/4 cup olive oil
- ✓ 2 garlic cloves, minced

Directions:

- ❖ In a grilling pan, cook the chicken breast until no longer pink or until a meat thermometer registers 5 degrees F. Slice the chicken into strips.
- ❖ Storing
- ❖ Place the chicken breasts in airtight containers or Ziploc bags; keep in your refrigerator for to 4 days.
- ❖ For freezing, place the chicken breasts in airtight containers or heavy-duty freezer bags. It will maintain the best quality for about months. Defrost in the refrigerator.
- ❖ Toss the chicken with the other ingredients. Prepare the dressing by whisking all the ingredients.
- ❖ Dress the salad and enjoy! Keep the salad in your refrigerator for 3 to 5 days.

Nutrition: 183 Calories; 12.5g Fat; 1. Carbs; 16.3g Protein; 0.9g Fiber

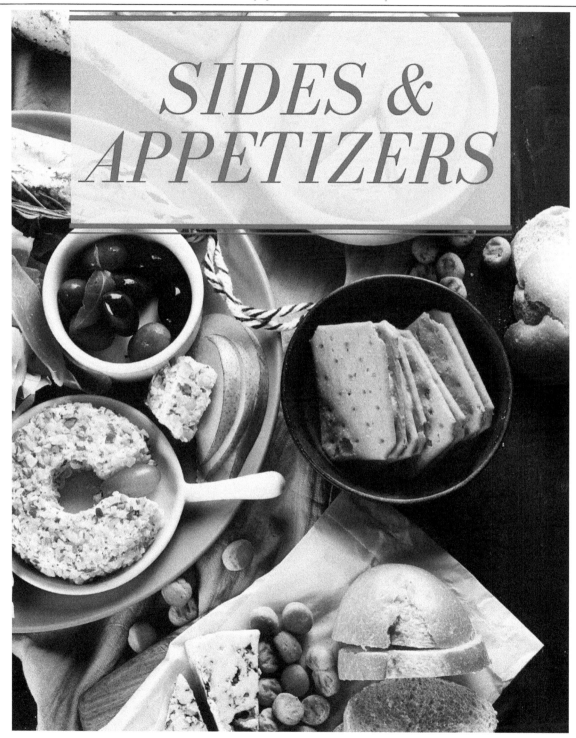

SIDES & APPETIZERS

92) TUSCAN BAKED MUSHROOMS

Cooking Time: 20 Minutes **Servings: 2**

Ingredients:
- ½ pound mushrooms (sliced)
- 2 tbsp olive oil (onion and garlic flavored)
- 1 can tomatoes
- 1 cup Parmesan cheese
- ½ tsp oregano
- 1 tbsp basil
- sea salt or plain salt
- freshly ground black pepper

Directions:
- ❖ Heat the olive oil in the pan and add the mushrooms, salt, and pepper. Cook for about 2 minutes.
- ❖ Then, transfer the mushrooms into a baking dish.
- ❖ Now, in a separate bowl mix the tomatoes, basil, oregano, salt, and pepper, and layer it on the mushrooms. Top it with Parmesan cheese.
- ❖ Finally, bake the dish at 0 degrees F for about 18-22 minutes or until done.
- ❖ Serve warm.

Nutrition: Calories: 358, Total Fat: 27 g, Saturated Fat: 10.2 g, Cholesterol: 40 mg, Sodium: 535 mg, Total Carbohydrate: 13 g, Dietary Fiber: 3.5 g, Total Sugars: 6.7 g, Protein: 23.2 g, Vitamin D: 408 mcg, Calcium: 526 mg, Iron: 4 mg, Potassium: 797 mg

93) TYPICAL MINT TABBOULEH

Cooking Time: 15 Minutes **Servings: 6**

Ingredients:
- ¼ cup fine bulgur
- 1/3 cup water, boiling
- 3 tbsp lemon juice
- ¼ tsp honey
- 1 1/3 cups pistachios, finely chopped
- 1 cup curly parsley, finely chopped
- 1 small cucumber, finely chopped
- 1 medium tomato, finely chopped
- 4 green onions, finely chopped
- 1/3 cup fresh mint, finely chopped
- 3 tbsp olive oil

Directions:
- ❖ Take a large bowl and add bulgur and 3 cup of boiling water.
- ❖ Allow it to stand for about 5 minutes.
- ❖ Stir in honey and lemon juice and allow it to stand for 5 minutes more.
- ❖ Fluff up the bulgur with a fork and stir in the rest of the Ingredients.
- ❖ Season with salt and pepper.
- ❖ Enjoy!

Nutrition: Calories: 15 Total Fat: 13.5 g, Saturated Fat: 1.8 g, Cholesterol: 0 mg, Sodium: 78 mg, Total Carbohydrate: 9.2 g, Dietary Fiber: 2.8 g, Total Sugars: 2.9 g, Protein: 3.8 g, Vitamin D: 0 mcg, Calcium: 46 mg, Iron: 2 mg, Potassium: 359 mg

94) Italian Scallops Pea Fettuccine

Cooking Time: 15 Minutes **Servings: 5**

Ingredients:
- 8 ounces whole-wheat fettuccine (pasta, macaroni)
- 1 pound large sea scallops
- ¼ tsp salt, divided
- 1 tbsp extra virgin olive oil
- 1 8-ounce bottle of clam juice
- 1 cup low-fat milk
- ¼ tsp ground white pepper
- 3 cups frozen peas, thawed
- ¾ cup finely shredded Romano cheese, divided
- 1/3 cup fresh chives, chopped
- ½ tsp freshly grated lemon zest
- 1 tsp lemon juice

Directions:
- ❖ Boil water in a large pot and cook fettuccine according to package instructions.
- ❖ Drain well and put it to the side.
- ❖ Heat oil in a large, non-stick skillet over medium-high heat.
- ❖ Pat the scallops dry and sprinkle them with 1/8 tsp of salt.
- ❖ Add the scallops to the skillet and cook for about 2-3 minutes per side until golden brown. Remove scallops from pan.
- ❖ Add clam juice to the pan you removed the scallops from.
- ❖ In another bowl, whisk in milk, white pepper, flour, and remaining 1/8 tsp of salt.
- ❖ Once the mixture is smooth, whisk into the pan with the clam juice.
- ❖ Bring the entire mix to a simmer and keep stirring for about 1-2 minutes until the sauce is thick.
- ❖ Return the scallops to the pan and add peas. Bring it to a simmer.
- ❖ Stir in fettuccine, chives, ½ a cup of Romano cheese, lemon zest, and lemon juice.
- ❖ Mix well until thoroughly combined.
- ❖ Cool and spread over containers.
- ❖ Before eating, serve with remaining cheese sprinkled on top.
- ❖ Enjoy!

Nutrition: Calories: 388, Total Fat: 9.2 g, Saturated Fat: 3.7 g, Cholesterol: 33 mg, Sodium: 645 mg, Total Carbohydrate: 50.1 g, Dietary Fiber: 10.4 g, Total Sugars: 8.7 g, Protein: 24.9 g, Vitamin D: 25 mcg, Calcium: 293 mg, Iron: 4 mg, Potassium: 247 mg

95) CLASSIC BASIL PASTA

Cooking Time: 40 Minutes   **Servings:** 4

Ingredients:

- ✓ 2 red peppers, de-seeded and cut into chunks
- ✓ 2 red onions cut into wedges
- ✓ 2 mild red chilies, de-seeded and diced
- ✓ 3 garlic cloves, coarsely chopped
- ✓ 1 tsp golden caster sugar
- ✓ 2 tbsp olive oil, plus extra for serving
- ✓ 2 pounds small ripe tomatoes, quartered
- ✓ 12 ounces pasta
- ✓ a handful of basil leaves, torn
- ✓ 2 tbsp grated parmesan
- ✓ salt
- ✓ pepper

Directions:

- ❖ Preheat oven to 390 degrees F.
- ❖ On a large roasting pan, spread peppers, red onion, garlic, and chilies.
- ❖ Sprinkle sugar on top.
- ❖ Drizzle olive oil and season with salt and pepper.
- ❖ Roast the veggies for 1minutes.
- ❖ Add tomatoes and roast for another 15 minutes.
- ❖ In a large pot, cook your pasta in salted boiling water according to instructions.
- ❖ Once ready, drain pasta.
- ❖ Remove the veggies from the oven and carefully add pasta.
- ❖ Toss everything well and let it cool.
- ❖ Spread over the containers.
- ❖ Before eating, place torn basil leaves on top, and sprinkle with parmesan.
- ❖ Enjoy!

Nutrition: Calories: 384, Total Fat: 10.8 g, Saturated Fat: 2.3 g, Cholesterol: 67 mg, Sodium: 133 mg, Total Carbohydrate: 59.4 g, Dietary Fiber: 2.3 g, Total Sugars: 5.7 g, Protein: 1 g, Vitamin D: 0 mcg, Calcium: 105 mg, Iron: 4 mg, Potassium: 422 mg

96) Veggie Mediterranean-style Pasta

Cooking Time: 2 Hours   **Servings:** 4

Ingredients:

- ✓ 1 tbsp olive oil
- ✓ 1 small onion, finely chopped
- ✓ 2 small garlic cloves, finely chopped
- ✓ 2 14-ounce cans diced tomatoes
- ✓ 1 tbsp sun-dried tomato paste
- ✓ 1 bay leaf
- ✓ 1 tsp dried thyme
- ✓ 1 tsp dried basil
- ✓ 1 tsp oregano
- ✓ 1 tsp dried parsley
- ✓ bread of your choice
- ✓ ½ tsp salt
- ✓ ½ tsp brown sugar
- ✓ freshly ground black pepper
- ✓ 1 piece aubergine
- ✓ 2 pieces courgettes
- ✓ 2 pieces red peppers, de-seeded
- ✓ 2 garlic cloves, peeled
- ✓ 2-3 tbsp olive oil
- ✓ 12 small vine-ripened tomatoes
- ✓ 16 ounces of pasta of your preferred shape, such as Gigli, conchiglie, etc.
- ✓ 3½ ounces parmesan cheese

Directions:

- ❖ Heat oil in a pan over medium heat.
- ❖ Add onions and fry them until tender.
- ❖ Add garlic and stir-fry for 1 minute.
- ❖ Add the remaining Ingredients: listed under the sauce and bring to a boil.
- ❖ Reduce the heat, cover, and simmer for 60 minutes.
- ❖ Season with black pepper and salt as needed. Set aside.
- ❖ Preheat oven to 350 degrees F.
- ❖ Chop up courgettes, aubergine and red peppers into 1-inch pieces.
- ❖ Place them on a roasting pan along with whole garlic cloves.
- ❖ Drizzle with olive oil and season with salt and black pepper.
- ❖ Mix the veggies well and roast in the oven for 45 minutes until they are tender.
- ❖ Add tomatoes just before 20 minutes to end time.
- ❖ Cook your pasta according to package instructions.
- ❖ Drain well and stir into the sauce.
- ❖ Divide the pasta sauce between 4 containers and top with vegetables.
- ❖ Grate some parmesan cheese on top and serve with bread.
- ❖ Enjoy!

Nutrition: Calories: 211, Total Fat: 14.9 g, Saturated Fat: 2.1 g, Cholesterol: 0 mg, Sodium: 317 mg, Total Carbohydrate: 20.1 g, Dietary Fiber: 5.7 g, Total Sugars: 11.7 g, Protein: 4.2 g, Vitamin D: 0 mcg, Calcium: 66 mg, Iron: 2 mg, Potassium: 955 mg

97) ORIGINAL RED ONION KALE PASTA

Cooking Time: 25 Minutes   **Servings: 4**

Ingredients:

- ✓ 2½ cups vegetable broth
- ✓ ¾ cup dry lentils
- ✓ ½ tsp of salt
- ✓ 1 bay leaf
- ✓ ¼ cup olive oil
- ✓ 1 large red onion, chopped
- ✓ 1 tsp fresh thyme, chopped
- ✓ ½ tsp fresh oregano, chopped

- ✓ 1 tsp salt, divided
- ✓ ½ tsp black pepper
- ✓ 8 ounces vegan sausage, sliced into ¼-inch slices
- ✓ 1 bunch kale, stems removed and coarsely chopped
- ✓ 1 pack rotini

Directions:

- ❖ Add vegetable broth, ½ tsp of salt, bay leaf, and lentils to a saucepan over high heat and bring to a boil.
- ❖ Reduce the heat to medium-low and allow to cook for about minutes until tender.
- ❖ Discard the bay leaf.
- ❖ Take another skillet and heat olive oil over medium-high heat.
- ❖ Stir in thyme, onions, oregano, ½ a tsp of salt, and pepper; cook for 1 minute.
- ❖ Add sausage and reduce heat to medium-low.
- ❖ Cook for 10 minutes until the onions are tender.
- ❖ Bring water to a boil in a large pot, and then add rotini pasta and kale.
- ❖ Cook for about 8 minutes until al dente.
- ❖ Remove a bit of the cooking water and put it to the side.
- ❖ Drain the pasta and kale and return to the pot.
- ❖ Stir in both the lentils mixture and the onions mixture.
- ❖ Add the reserved cooking liquid to add just a bit of moistness.
- ❖ Spread over containers.

Nutrition: Calories: 508, Total Fat: 17 g, Saturated Fat: 3 g, Cholesterol: 0 mg, Sodium: 2431 mg, Total Carbohydrate: 59.3 g, Dietary Fiber: 6 g, Total Sugars: 4.8 g, Protein: 30.9 g, Vitamin D: 0 mcg, Calcium: 256 mg, Iron: 8 mg, Potassium: 1686 mg

98) Special Braised Artichokes

Cooking Time: 30 Minutes   **Servings: 6**

Ingredients:

- ✓ 6 tbsp olive oil
- ✓ 2 pounds baby artichokes, trimmed
- ✓ ½ cup lemon juice
- ✓ 4 garlic cloves, thinly sliced

- ✓ ½ tsp salt
- ✓ 1½ pounds tomatoes, seeded and diced
- ✓ ½ cup almonds, toasted and sliced

Directions:

- ❖ Heat oil in a skillet over medium heat.
- ❖ Add artichokes, garlic, and lemon juice, and allow the garlic to sizzle.
- ❖ Season with salt.
- ❖ Reduce heat to medium-low, cover, and simmer for about 15 minutes.
- ❖ Uncover, add tomatoes, and simmer for another 10 minutes until the tomato liquid has mostly evaporated.
- ❖ Season with more salt and pepper.
- ❖ Sprinkle with toasted almonds.
- ❖ Enjoy!

Nutrition: Calories: 265, Total Fat: 1g, Saturated Fat: 2.6 g, Cholesterol: 0 mg, Sodium: 265 mg, Total Carbohydrate: 23 g, Dietary Fiber: 8.1 g, Total Sugars: 12.4 g, Protein: 7 g, Vitamin D: 0 mcg, Calcium: 81 mg, Iron: 2 mg, Potassium: 1077 mg

99) DELICIOUS FRIED GREEN BEANS

Cooking Time: 15 Minutes   **Servings: 2**

Ingredients:

- ✓ ½ pound green beans, trimmed
- ✓ 1 egg
- ✓ 2 tbsp olive oil
- ✓ 1¼ tbsp almond flour

- ✓ 2 tbsp parmesan cheese
- ✓ ½ tsp garlic powder
- ✓ sea salt or plain salt
- ✓ freshly ground black pepper

Directions:

- ❖ Start by beating the egg and olive oil in a bowl.
- ❖ Then, mix the remaining Ingredients: in a separate bowl and set aside.
- ❖ Now, dip the green beans in the egg mixture and then coat with the dry mix.
- ❖ Finally, grease a baking pan, then transfer the beans to the pan and bake at 5 degrees F for about 12-15 minutes or until crisp.
- ❖ Serve warm.

Nutrition: Calories: 334, Total Fat: 23 g, Saturated Fat: 8.3 g, Cholesterol: 109 mg, Sodium: 397 mg, Total Carbohydrate: 10.9 g, Dietary Fiber: 4.3 g, Total Sugars: 1.9 g, Protein: 18.1 g, Vitamin D: 8 mcg, Calcium: 398 mg, Iron: 2 mg, Potassium: 274 mg

100) ARTICHOKE OLIVE PASTA

Cooking Time: 25 Minutes   **Servings: 4**

Ingredients:
- ✓ salt
- ✓ pepper
- ✓ 2 tbsp olive oil, divided
- ✓ 2 garlic cloves, thinly sliced
- ✓ 1 can artichoke hearts, drained, rinsed, and quartered lengthwise
- ✓ 1-pint grape tomatoes, halved lengthwise, divided
- ✓ ½ cup fresh basil leaves, torn apart
- ✓ 12 ounces whole-wheat spaghetti
- ✓ ½ medium onion, thinly sliced
- ✓ ½ cup dry white wine
- ✓ 1/3 cup pitted Kalamata olives, quartered lengthwise
- ✓ ¼ cup grated Parmesan cheese, plus extra for serving

Directions:
- ❖ Fill a large pot with salted water.
- ❖ Pour the water to a boil and cook your pasta according to package instructions until al dente.
- ❖ Drain the pasta and reserve 1 cup of the cooking water.
- ❖ Return the pasta to the pot and set aside.
- ❖ Heat 1 tbsp of olive oil in a large skillet over medium-high heat.
- ❖ Add onion and garlic, season with pepper and salt, and cook well for about 3-4 minutes until nicely browned.
- ❖ Add wine and cook for 2 minutes until evaporated.
- ❖ Stir in artichokes and keep cooking 2-3 minutes until brown.
- ❖ Add olives and half of your tomatoes.
- ❖ Cook well for 1-2 minutes until the tomatoes start to break down.
- ❖ Add pasta to the skillet.
- ❖ Stir in the rest of the tomatoes, cheese, basil, and remaining oil.
- ❖ Thin the mixture with the reserved pasta water if needed.
- ❖ Place in containers and sprinkle with extra cheese.
- ❖ Enjoy!

Nutrition: 340, Total Fat: 11.9 g, Saturated Fat: 3.3 g, Cholesterol: 10 mg, Sodium: 278 mg, Total Carbohydrate: 35.8 g, Dietary Fiber: 7.8 g, Total Sugars: 4.8 g, Protein: 11.6 g, Vitamin D: 0 mcg, Calcium: 193 mg, Iron: 3 mg, Potassium: 524 mg

101) MEDITERRANEAN OLIVE TUNA PASTA

Cooking Time: 20 Minutes   **Servings: 4**

Ingredients:
- ✓ 8 ounces of tuna steak, cut into 3 pieces
- ✓ ¼ cup green olives, chopped
- ✓ 3 cloves garlic, minced
- ✓ 2 cups grape tomatoes, halved
- ✓ ½ cup white wine
- ✓ 2 tbsp lemon juice
- ✓ 6 ounces pasta - whole wheat gobetti, rotini, or penne
- ✓ 1 10-ounce package frozen artichoke hearts, thawed and squeezed dry
- ✓ 4 tbsp extra-virgin olive oil, divided
- ✓ 2 tsp fresh grated lemon zest
- ✓ 2 tsp fresh rosemary, chopped, divided
- ✓ ½ tsp salt, divided
- ✓ ¼ tsp fresh ground pepper
- ✓ ¼ cup fresh basil, chopped

Directions:
- ❖ Preheat grill to medium-high heat.
- ❖ Take a large pot of water and put it on to boil.
- ❖ Place the tuna pieces in a bowl and add 1 tbsp of oil, 1 tsp of rosemary, lemon zest, a ¼ tsp of salt, and pepper.
- ❖ Grill the tuna for about 3 minutes per side.
- ❖ Transfer tuna to a plate and allow it to cool.
- ❖ Place the pasta in boiling water and cook according to package instructions.
- ❖ Drain the pasta.
- ❖ Flake the tuna into bite-sized pieces.
- ❖ In a large skillet, heat remaining oil over medium heat.
- ❖ Add artichoke hearts, garlic, olives, and remaining rosemary.
- ❖ Cook for about 3-4 minutes until slightly browned.
- ❖ Add tomatoes, wine, and bring the mixture to a boil.
- ❖ Cook for about 3 minutes until the tomatoes are broken down.
- ❖ Stir in pasta, lemon juice, tuna, and remaining salt.
- ❖ Cook for 1-2 minutes until nicely heated.
- ❖ Spread over the containers.
- ❖ Before eating, garnish with some basil and enjoy!

Nutrition: 455, Total Fat: 21.2 g, Saturated Fat: 3.5 g, Cholesterol: 59 mg, Sodium: 685 mg, Total Carbohydrate: 38.4 g, Dietary Fiber: 6.1 g, Total Sugars: 3.5 g, Protein: 25.5 g, Vitamin D: 0 mcg, Calcium: 100 mg, Iron: 5 mg, Potassium: 800 mg

CONCLUSIONS

Today, we desire most is neither money nor lavish mansions, but the happiness of living a healthy life. Moreover, we are ready to pay any price for that and equally ready to follow any workout routine. It is a fact that there is a direct relationship between our fitness and the food we eat. If that food is more plant-based and has good monosaturated fats along with protein, it is a blessing. If it's time-tested, it's even better. This is what we find in the Mediterranean diet. Going through all these everyday diet recipes - breakfast, lunch, dinner, and snacks - it becomes clear that there is no room for unhealthy fats, preservatives, refined sugar, or flour. All of these foods tax different systems in our bodies. Plus, the diet doesn't burn a hole in your pocket, and the ingredients are readily available.

At first, it may be challenging to switch entirely to the Mediterranean diet. As they say, change is always tricky. You can do this at first by swapping any meal of the day: breakfast, lunch, dinner, or even snacks. This diet will make you feel light and healthy, both physically and mentally. This is an input that keeps us on track as we follow this diet. By only doing cardio, you may not be able to save your heart healthy. A reduced amount of weight would mean a lower chance of type 2 diabetes.

You notice in all the recipes in the diet of people living in the Mediterranean basin that it has plants or fish. This means it has healthy meat and all-natural ingredients with protein, micronutrients, and fiber that make our internal biological system work well. The fiber helps clean our internal system, while the chickpea, which is rich in vitamin D and has calcium, is also rich in calcium. Similarly, fruits such as banana, avocado, sweet potato; vegetables such as tomato, spinach, broccoli, ginger, mushroom, and garlic; and dried fruits such as pistachio currant. As for fats, there are only healthy ones that come from olive oil. Also, wheat and whole grains keep you conscious of being full and allow you to manage cravings. The good news is that many options and recipes resemble the items that decorate our plates today: pizza, muffins, salads, snacks, pitas, yogurt, sauces, etc. Besides, you can easily choose between vegan, vegetarian and non-vegetarian. This shows that following the Mediterranean diet is easy, even in the long run. But you have to start doing it.

Thank you for reading this book

Alexander Sandler